Healing Chair Yoga
for Every Body

by Linda Anastasia Ransom

The content of this book is a synthesis of the author's training and experience, and is not a substitute for professional medical advice, diagnosis, or treatment. Please seek advice from your healthcare provider for your personal health concerns prior to undertaking a new healthcare regimen as presented in this book. The author, illustrator, editor, publisher, and distributor assume no responsibility or liability for any injuries or losses that may result from practicing healing chair yoga.

Illustrated by Phillip Timper

Library of Congress Control Number: 2023907888
ISBN: 979-8-218-17321-0

Printed in the United States of America

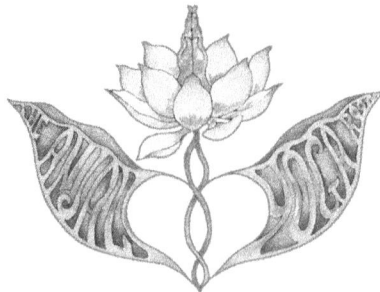

Wellness Within
1400 East Bogard Road
Wasilla, Alaska 99654
healingchairyoga@gmail.com

For all the teachers and students
of The Anjali Yoga Room,
their beautiful essence

Praise for Healing Chair Yoga with Linda Anastasia Ransom

Healing Chair Yoga is a beautiful experience, available to all, that quiets the mind and heals the body.
~Suzanne C.

One of the beautiful things about Healing Chair Yoga is the opportunity for anyone to practice yoga. Most of the yoga poses can be done in a chair. It's so beneficial for the healing of the body, and it's lovely that people who have issues with getting up and down can reap the powerful effects of yoga. It's especially wonderful if you have Linda as your teacher.
~Kath W.

Healing Chair Yoga was a lifeline. It proved that my body can move, stretch, and be strengthened!
~Roberta R.

I'm smiling more, and I even practice Mountain Pose and Tree Pose in line at the grocery store. Healing Chair Yoga has changed my life!
~Mary D.

Healing Chair Yoga is just that: healing, for one's mind, body, and spirit. Linda is a kind, supportive, and encouraging instructor. She creates a safe and welcoming space to heal.
~Susan C.

Healing Chair Yoga was a godsend. I came out of cancer radiation treatment and into Healing Chair Yoga and continued for five years. It helped me gain my mental and physical energy back and center my emotions, and I became a better person for it.
~Kat L.

I started taking Healing Chair Yoga, and amazing things happened. I felt more relaxed and could breathe again. My blood pressure even went down!
~Julie S.

Walking into a Healing Chair Yoga class is like walking into a private forest! Everyone is there for the same purpose: release the old and bring in the new. Calm and easy flowing movements open up your heart and soul and set you on the correct path for the rest of your day.
~Liz S.

Healing Chair Yoga is gentle and easy to follow; and, with my disability, it helps me maintain muscle tone and posture.
~Nikki R.

Healing Chair Yoga has made it possible for me to feel normal again with the nerve damage in my leg. Being part of a class with laughter and, most of all, love is a spiritual and physical healing. Stretching and breathing right empowers my body as well as my heart.
~Mary S.

Healing Chair Yoga and Linda's beautiful, loving spirit have enriched my life in so many ways. Even when I'm not able to attend a class, I can stand in Tree Pose and again experience all the wonderful, positive, caring energy I do love.
~Sharon S.

A surgeon said I'm a candidate for double-hip replacement, but I didn't want to go that route. A friend brought me to Healing Chair Yoga class, and I diligently came to class every week after that. Much to my surprise, a year later I had no pain in my hips, I was walking normally, and my flexibility returned.
~Linda R.

I so enjoyed the new movements my body really needed to heal! This gentle yoga is so forgiving.
~Ann M.

True mindfulness is gratitude.
~Linda Anastasia Ransom

Acknowledgments

My deepest gratitude to an extraordinary teacher, Lynne Minton, trained by B.K.S. Iyengar, for her guidance, expertise, and encouragement in pursuing my dream to write this book. Lynne led me through my RYT-200 (2006) and RYT-500 training (2015–2016), with the utmost thoroughness and precision.

A special thank-you to Lonnie Chace for training me, during my RYT-200, in teaching Healing Chair Yoga to cancer patients. I am also forever grateful to my other primary teachers, Sarahjoy Marsh, Alison Till, Dori McDannold, and Tammy Moser.

My deepest gratitude, also, to Sharon Story, dear friend and fellow yogi in my RYT-500 training. Sharon and I decided to fulfill our Final Master Project-Thesis together, by writing blogs about Healing Chair Yoga for the website of The Anjali Yoga Room. Along with our blog editor, Lindsey Kanter, we dreamed of eventually compiling that content into a book, though decided we were satisfied with what we'd achieved with the blog format.

In June 2021, during the COVID-19 pandemic, I dedicated myself to finally writing this book, with a renewed purpose to share the therapeutic benefits of yoga for all bodies. Sharon gave me her blessing to be this book's sole author, to re-create it in alignment with my vision.

Sixteen years after my first Healing Chair Yoga training, *Healing Chair Yoga for Every Body* is here, in your hands! A humble thank-you to you for trusting me to guide you through these pages.

A big thank-you to the book's production team: my editor, Marj Hahne, with the biggest hug of gratitude for your knowledge and patience; my graphic designer, Phillip Timper; and my blog/website designer, Nancy Timper.

A special thank-you to the models behind the book's images: my sisters, Bobbi Ransom-Rheaume and Nikki Ransom, and my dear friends Suzanne Crosby and Kathy Widmer. A huge thank-you to my husband, Bob Cederholm; my son, Nico Ransom Cederholm; and my future daughter in-law, Nikki McNutt, for taking photo after photo and for assisting me with computer technology. Of course, I thank my dog, Dave, who wanted to be in every picture taken for this book!

My heart is overflowing with heartfelt appreciation for all.

With love and gratitude. Namaste,
Linda Anastasia Ransom

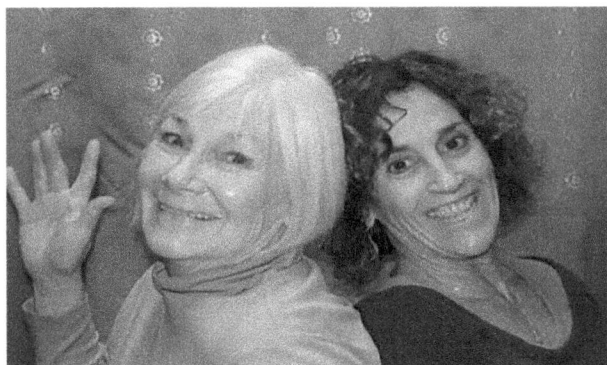

Sharon and Linda

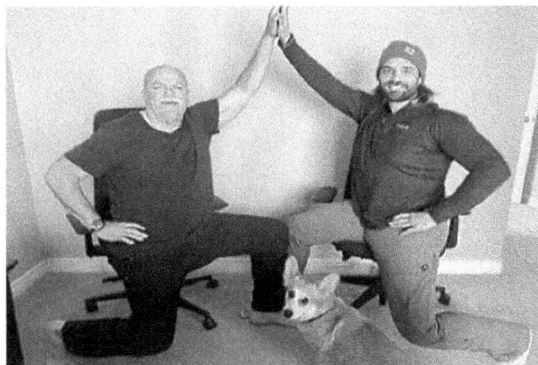

Bob, Dave, and Nico

Every yoga class is a beginning.
~Linda Anastasia Ransom

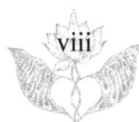

Table of Contents

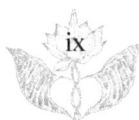

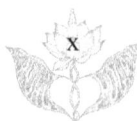

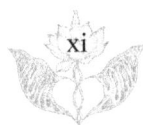

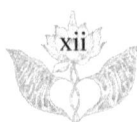

CHAPTER I

Introduction: What Is Yoga?

atha yogānuśāsanam
"And now, the practice of yoga begins."
~Patañjali

Is Healing Chair Yoga the same as yoga? Yes, of course! Just add a chair!

Yoga means "to yoke or unite." Yoga originated in India over 5000 years ago as a system of physical, mental, and spiritual development. This healing tool helps us rebalance the physical, mental, emotional, and spiritual aspects of our being so that we can feel whole rather than fragmented and unsettled. Yoga teaches us how to quiet the mind and live harmoniously in our body and in the world. Yoga is not a religion, but it can deepen and expand our spiritual journey, asking us to live with awareness, integrity, and compassion for all creation.

Physical yoga is known as Hatha yoga. Hatha (ha-tha) yoga is a practice grounded in the eight limbs of yoga: *asana* (physical postures), *pranayama* (breathing exercises), *yama* (rules of moral code), *niyama* (rules of personal behavior), *pratyahara* (withdrawal of the senses), *dharana* (concentration), *dhyana* (meditation), and *samadhi* (complete integration).

The physical postures help us observe, balance, and bring together the body and mind with the breath. Our health is reclaimed and maintained, the emotions are stabilized, and the mind becomes more peaceful. Hatha yoga allows us the opportunity to express ourselves from the inside out.

"We are not here to change ourselves. We are here to meet ourselves where we are." In the spirit of this yogic saying, let's start our journey of self-discovery from where we are and go from there.

Common Questions for Beginners

Do I have to be flexible to do yoga?
No. Yoga creates flexibility of mind and body. It's not required that you already be limber in order to participate. Yoga is a science of mind as well as body.

What type of physical condition do I need to be in to practice yoga?
Anyone can practice the physical postures of yoga. There is a beginning asana for everyone. Check with your physician before beginning any exercise program, especially if you have any

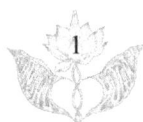

condition or injury, and talk to your yoga teacher about what classes may be the best fit for you. We want your practice to be appropriate and healthful for your body.

What if I am pregnant or have a medical condition?

Consult your doctor before starting, or returning to, any physical activity. Particularly if you are pregnant or have high blood pressure or glaucoma, consult your doctor before adding inversions to your yoga practice—poses in which the heart is higher from the ground than the head.

What should I wear?

Wear comfortable workout clothes: shorts, leggings, or sweatpants; a tank top or T-shirt; no shoes or socks unless necessary for balance. Yoga is done in bare feet.

How often do I need to practice yoga?

At least three times a week is recommended, but if you work consistently with a balanced set of postures, your progress will be realized on many fronts: mental, physical, spiritual, some unexpected. All you need is commitment plus a playful sense of observation and experimentation.

What equipment do I need?

Yoga can be done on a mat or a chair; in Healing Chair Yoga, we use both, with props—blocks, a strap, and bolsters—for assistance. You may purchase yoga accessories or fashion your own. A small stack of hardcover books or wood can serve as a block. For a strap, use a scarf or tie. Sturdy pillows, towels, and blankets make great bolsters. Be creative! You don't have to spend lots of money.

What are the benefits of yoga?

Numerous and manifold! Yoga has been proven to be more beneficial—physiologically, psychologically, biochemically—than regular exercise.

Physiological benefits:
- Increases energy, stamina, and endurance
- Increases immunity
- Improves sleep
- Improves physical strength and balance
- Decreases pain levels
- Decreases blood pressure, pulse rate, and respiratory rate
- Improves cardiovascular, respiratory, endocrinal, and gastrointestinal functioning
- Increases flexibility and joint efficiency
- Improves reactive responses and eye-hand coordination

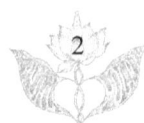

Psychological benefits:
- Improves mood and well-being
- Decreases anxiety and depression
- Improves concentration and attention span
- Improves memory, cognition, and perception

Biochemical benefits:
- Decreases glucose, sodium, and cholesterol levels
- Increases thyroxine and vitamin-C levels

Now that we've covered the *what* of Healing Chair Yoga, let's move on to the *how*.

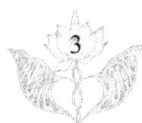

Yoga is the breath within the breath.
~Linda Anastasia Ransom

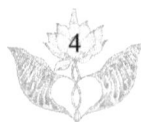

CHAPTER II

The Internal Workings of Yoga: Alignment, Pranayama, Mudras, Mantras, and Meditation

Healing Chair Yoga, like all yoga, deepens our moment-by-moment experience of this human journey. In this chapter, you will learn proper alignment and a variety of breathing techniques (pranayama), hand positions (mudras), sacred sounds (mantras), and meditations to relax the body and quiet the mind. You may do these practices separately or integrate them into your yoga practice.

With its creative use of props, Healing Chair Yoga allows for adaptability to your moment-by-moment physical needs. Blocks extend our limbs; bolsters bring the ground to the body. Props assist with stability, release, and relaxation; some allow modification of, or progression in, a pose.

Props needed:
- A sturdy chair and a yoga mat
- 2 blocks (purchased or constructed 8″x 6″x 4″)
- A yoga strap, scarf, or tie
- 2 bolsters or study pillows
- 2–4 blankets or bath towels

Tadasana Alignment

Alignment creates a steady base for a safe yoga practice. Alignment allows the body, seated or standing, to stretch and open while reducing wear and tear on the joints and tissues, bringing ease and grace to your practice. Maintain alignment during every asana, pranayama, and meditation. Alignment is also a life tool for good posture and renewed health: maintain it in your daily life, when you're driving, eating a meal, waiting in line. Your body wants to be healthy and happy all the time.

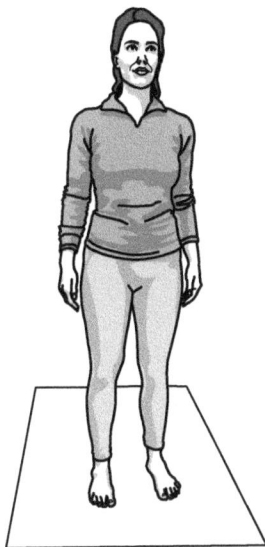

1. Begin with your feet:
   a. Standing: Place your feet on the mat, hip-width apart, such that your ankles are directly below the knees.
   Seated: Place a blanket under the feet, if

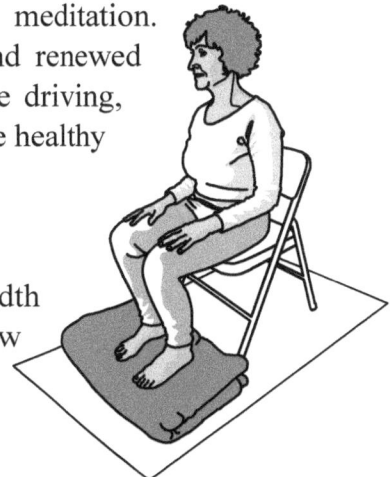

needed, to align the knees with the hips. Always place a mat under your chair for stability and safety.

    b. Spread your toes.

    c. Press the mound of your big toes into the mat, then the pinky toes, the remaining toes, the inside of the heels, and the outside of the heels.

2. Engage your core:
    a. Bring the energy up from the earth through your toes, lower legs, knees, and thighs, to your pelvic bowl, your core center.
    b. Bring your belly in and up.

3. Align the rest of your body.
    a. Bring your shoulders back and down, and relax your arms and hands at your sides, if standing; or, if seated, place your palms on your lap, faceup to receive energy or facedown for grounding.
    b. Keeping your chin parallel to the floor, press your nose to the back of the skull.
    c. Imagine a string attached to the crown of your head, lengthening you toward the sky.

4. Feel the grounding energy from your soles to the crown of your head.

Do you feel taller now? This is Healing Chair Yoga alignment—Tadasana, or Mountain Pose—the foundation for correct alignment in all asanas.

Pranayama

Prana means "breath, vital energy, life force"; *yama* means "to control or maintain." Pranayama, then, is the process of controlling and maintaining the breath, vital energy, and life force. Though learning the depths and nuanced techniques of pranayama through consistent practice can take years, its basic techniques bring immediate benefits[1] to new practitioners:

- Quiets the mind, improving the mind-body connection
- Stabilizes the emotions, lessening reactivity
- Expands awareness in the present moment
- Reduces physiological and psycho-emotional stress
- Lowers heart rate and improves cardiovascular functioning
- Improves lung functioning and respiratory endurance
- Regulates the autonomic nervous system, which controls our respiration, heartbeat, digestion, and more. Its two parts—the sympathetic nervous system and the parasympathetic nervous system—are responsible, respectively, for our fight-or-flight response and our resting response.

Only 90 seconds of pranayama can calm our activated thoughts and emotions, centering us, grounding us. We breathe 20,000 to 22,000 breaths daily. How many of us are aware of just one breath?

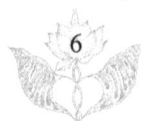

As you work through the following breathing techniques, please be gentle and patient with yourself; this journey is a practice, not perfection. If you would like to explore a deeper practice beyond what's offered here, we recommend working with an experienced teacher.

Below are seven types of pranayama to explore, one per sitting. As a new yogi, practice these techniques for no more than two to three minutes each, using a timer if you like. Over time, you can work your way to increasingly longer practice times.

Precaution: If, at any time during your practice, you start to feel uncomfortable or agitated, or your breath becomes strained, stop and return to natural breathing. Take a moment, and, when you feel inspired to do so, begin again. You may start and stop as many times as you need to; over time, your discomfort should decrease. The objective is to help you become calm and centered.

Observing the Breath and Setting an Intention

1. Breathe through your nostrils.
2. Observe your normal breath as it flows in and out.
3. Start a silent metronome in your mind, roughly one beat per second.
4. Count how many beats it takes to inhale, and how many beats to exhale.
5. Even out the length of your inhalations and exhalations by gently expanding whichever is shorter.
6. Eventually let go of the counting and continue the breathing pattern naturally.
7. Notice how your body and mind are feeling after several more breaths.
8. You can add an intention with any pranayama: inhale "I am," and exhale your desired state of being (e.g., "safe," "healthy," "lovable," "perfect as I am"). Your intention can be a scripted mantra (p. 13).

Breathing in, I calm my body. Breathing out, I smile.
Dwelling in the present moment I know this is a wonderful moment.
~Thich Nhat Hanh, *Being Peace*[2]

Opening Your Pranayama Practice

As you learn the seven pranayamas that follow, keep your practice short and steady. Start with one to two minutes, eventually working up to three to five minutes if you still feel refreshed. If you ever feel lightheaded, stop and return to your normal breath. Always be kind and loving to yourself.

1. Find a comfortable, peaceful place, sitting on either a chair or a mat on the floor. Position your body:
   a. Chair: Prop a bolster or block, if needed, vertically from the sacrum, along your spine, and sit so that your feet are on the floor, ankles vertically aligned

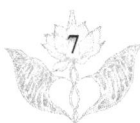

with the knees. Roll your shoulders back and down, keeping your chin parallel to the floor. To keep your knees horizontally aligned with the hips, you may need to place a folded blanket under your feet.

    b. Mat: Sit (on a bolster or blanket if needed), your back erect and your legs cross-legged (with a block under each knee if needed). If your body needs more support, lean against a wall, with or without a bolster or block propped vertically from the sacrum, along your spine. Roll your shoulders back and down, keeping your chin parallel to the floor. (If your body needs to recline, you may lie on your back with a bolster or blanket under the knees and a blanket or towel under your head and neck folded thin enough to maintain the natural curvature of your neck.)

2. Position your palms:
    a. Chair: Place palms on your lap, facing upward for receiving energy or downward for grounding.
    b. Mat: Place palms on your lap if sitting, at your sides if lying down, facing upward for receiving energy or downward for grounding.

3. Check in with your body to make sure your head, neck, back, and limbs are warm and comfortable and in alignment. Breathe naturally, and let your mind and body relax.

"Ha" Pranayama

This technique can be done before your yoga practice or anytime during the day when you want to let go of what no longer serves you.

1. Inhale slowly through the nostrils, expanding the belly.
2. Exhale slowly through the mouth with an audible "haaaa," contracting the belly.
3. Breathe for three breaths as a preliminary to another pranayama technique, or continue for one to three minutes.

Ujjayi Pranayama
"victorious breath," ocean-like breath

This breath, one of the first we learn in yoga, is generally used in most asanas. It can be done anytime, anywhere: working at your computer, listening on the phone, standing in line at the grocery store. Audible and powerful, it's also referred to as the "Darth Vader breath"!

1. Inhale and exhale slowly, softly, evenly through the nostrils.
2. Inhale through the nostrils, bringing the breath up through the rib cage and into the two lobes of the lungs, making a whispering "ah" sound with lips closed.
3. Exhale through the nostrils, from the back of your throat, creating a soft sound of crashing waves, or making a "ha" sound with lips closed.
4. Continue for two to three minutes, then come back to your normal breath.

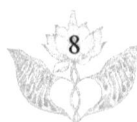

Dirga Pranayama
"complete," three-part breath

For this technique, we actively breathe into three parts of the torso—belly, rib cage, and chest—either sitting in a chair or lying on a mat (the latter will allow you to feel the breath moving uninterrupted through your body). This breath can release anxiety and panic attacks.

1. Complete three "Ha" breaths (p. 8).
2. Inhale, expanding the belly like a balloon.
3. Exhale through the nostrils, drawing the navel towards the spine to release all the air from the belly.
4. Inhale through the nostrils, filling the belly with air. When the belly is full, sip in a little more air to expand into the rib cage, widening apart the ribs, and then bring the air to your upper chest, your heart center.
5. Exhale through the nostrils, reversing the flow of breath, releasing it first from the upper chest such that the heart center sinks, then from the rib cage such that the ribs slide closer together, and then from the low belly, drawing the navel back towards the spine.
6. Continue for three to five breaths. To develop a fluid wave of air up and down the torso, place one hand, successively with the breath, in each of the three positions—the belly just below the navel, the lower half of the rib cage, the chest just above the sternum, and then the reverse—to feel the air moving in and out of each, eventually relaxing your effort.
7. Variation: Inhale as in #4, but for the exhale, release the air first from the belly, then from the rib cage, then from the chest, which may create a deeper relaxation response.
8. Choosing the variation that feels best for you, continue for three to five minutes, then come back to your normal breath.

Sama Vritti Pranayama
"equal rotation/flow," box or square breathing

Sama means "same"; *vritti* means "fluctuations of mind"—that is, equal inhalations and exhalations bringing peace to the busy mind. This technique is used by the Navy SEALs to reduce stress response and thus reduce sleep time.

1. Inhale and exhale slowly through the nostrils.
2. Inhale for a slow count of four, pause, and hold the breath for a count of four.
3. Exhale for a slow count of four, pause, and hold the breath for a count of four.
4. Continue for three to five minutes, then come back to your normal breath.

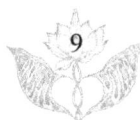

Viloma I Pranayama

This technique—an interrupted-inhalation practice where one pauses several times while inhaling—is said to increase energy and mitigate low blood pressure. It is typically practiced in the morning to get the day off to a good start, but it can be done at any time of day.

1. Inhale and exhale slowly and fully through the nostrils.
2. Inhale for a slow count of six, pause, and exhale for a slow count of six.
3. Once this pattern is set, inhale for counts one and two, pause, inhale for counts three and four, pause, inhale for counts five and six, pause, then exhale slowly and fully.
4. Inhale one-two, pause, inhale three-four, pause, inhale five-six, pause, exhale slowly and fully.
5. Continue for two to three minutes, then come back to your normal breath.

Don't worry if you can't inhale or exhale for the full six counts right away. Remember to return to your natural breathing whenever you need to, then begin again.

Viloma II Pranayama

This technique—an interrupted-exhalation practice where one pauses several times while exhaling—is said to quiet the mind and mitigate high blood pressure. Though typically practiced in the evening to promote restful sleep, it can be practiced at any time of day.

1. Inhale and exhale slowly and fully through the nostrils.
2. Inhale for a slow count of six, pause, and exhale for a slow count of six.
3. Once this pattern is set, inhale for a slow count of six, exhale for counts one and two, pause, exhale for counts three and four, pause, exhale for counts five and six, and pause.
4. Inhale slowly and fully, exhale one-two, pause, exhale three-four, pause, exhale five-six, and pause.
5. Continue for two to three minutes, then come back to your normal breath.

Don't worry if you can't inhale or exhale for the full six counts right away. Remember to return to your natural breathing whenever you need to, then begin again.

Nadi Shodhana Pranayama
"channel purification," alternate-nostril breathing

This technique clears the foggy mind by balancing the brain's right and left hemispheres.

1. Place your left hand on your left thigh.
2. Close the right nostril with your right thumb, bringing your index and middle fingers to the base of the thumb, and exhale completely.

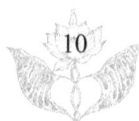

3. Inhale through the left nostril, then close the left nostril with your right ring-finger.
4. Open the right nostril, and exhale through this nostril.
5. Inhale through the right nostril, then close this nostril with your right thumb.
6. Open the left nostril, and exhale through this nostril to complete one cycle.
7. Continue for three to five minutes (or less time if that feels better), always completing this practice with an exhalation on the left side.

Completing Your Pranayama Practice

1. Position your body:
   a. Chair: Place your palms facing upward or downward on your lap, and come back to your normal breath.
   b. Mat: Lie on your mat quietly for a moment. Roll onto your right side, stretching your right arm under your head, and stay for a few breaths. Slowly press yourself up to a comfortable seated position.

2. Bring your palms together at your heart, bow your head, and say *Namaste* aloud or silently to show respect for that which is good in all beings.

Mudras

Mudra means "seal, mark, or gesture"—that is, a gesture or position, usually performed with the hands and fingers, that acts as "a lock" to guide energy flow and reflexes to the brain during your pranayama, meditation, and yoga practice.

Used for thousands of years, mudras are an outward representation of your inward intentions. Meditating on a specific mudra below will help you clarify and manifest a certain hope, energy, or devotion into your life. More than 400 mudras have been mentioned in different texts and by different yogis, but here are several foundational ones:

Anjali or Namaste Mudra
Mudra of Divine Offering and Respect

- Placement: Place the palms together in front of the chest.
- Benefits: Offers reverence and respect for differences; humbles oneself; surrenders oneself to the beauty of life.

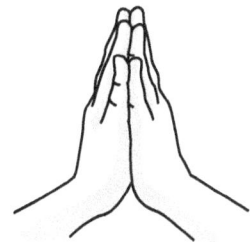

Gyan Mudra
Mudra of Knowledge and Wisdom

- Placement: Touch the tip of the thumbs to the tip of the index fingers.
- Benefits: Facilitates inner strength, self-worth, confidence, wisdom, higher self-knowledge, love, unity with one's chosen divine being.

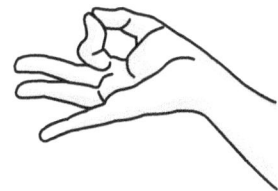

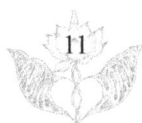

Shuni Mudra
Mudra of the Seal of Patience
- Placement: Touch the tip of the thumbs to the tip of the middle fingers.
- Benefits: Facilitates patience, responsibility, balance; calms emotions; promotes discernment and commitment.

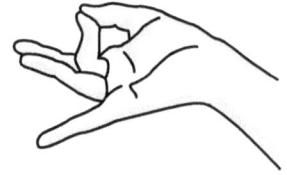

Surya Mudra
Mudra of the Sun and Earth
- Placement: Touch the tip of the thumbs to the tip of the ring fingers.
- Benefits: Balances the physical body, health, life energy, relationship to others and family; helps one find trust and security; helps one adjust to a life change or disruption.

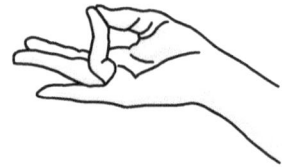

Buddhi Mudra
Mudra of Liquid and Flowing Systems of the Body
- Placement: Touch the tip of the thumbs to the tip of the pinky fingers.
- Benefits: Promotes communication, inner calmness, creativity; elevates mood; helps one discern intuitive messages; purifies the kidneys and adrenal glands; balances the water element in the body; activates the salivary glands; provides moisture to the skin and eyes.

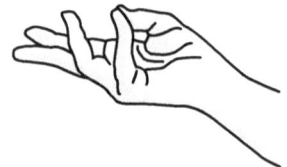

Abhaya Mudra
Mudra of Fearlessness, Protection, and Peace
- Placement: Make a Stop gesture with the right hand only.
- Benefits: Facilitates positive energy, as one lets go of fear, panic, anxiety, phobias, all negative energy.

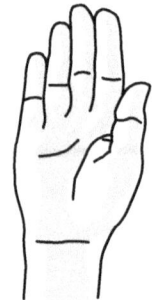

Mantras

Mantra means "sacred sound"—that is, a syllable, word, or phrase you may repeat, either aloud or silently, during your pranayama, meditation, or yoga practice. By giving you something to focus on, a mantra helps minimize distracting thoughts.

Choose a scripted mantra (p. 13) or a simple word or phrase expressing a desired behavior (e.g., breathe, let go) or an intended state of being (e.g., peace, calm, confidence, love), in which case, add "in" on the inhale (e.g., "Peace in.") and "out" on the exhale (e.g., "Peace out."). Repeat the mantra softly, gently, whether aloud or silently, as many times as you need to quiet the mind. Allow the breath to fall away into its own rhythm. As you sink more deeply into a meditative state, quieting the mind, the mantra becomes effortless and eventually dissolves.

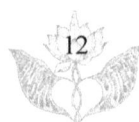

"Om" Mantra

Om (or *Aum*) is said to be the sacred sound of the universe, the sound we hear in utero, the sound of the wind, the rain, the ocean, the mountain brooks. It represents the divine within you. Om is traditionally chanted three times at the beginning or end of a yoga practice, releasing negativity and bringing calm and positive energy to the mind and body.

1. Inhale slowly through the nostrils.
2. Exhale, pronouncing the first syllable as "ah," the second syllable as "oo," and the third syllable as "mm."

"All Is Well" Mantra

This sequence affirms the perfection of the present, past, and future.

1. Inhale "All is well."
2. Exhale "All was well."
3. Inhale "All shall be well."
4. Exhale the breath slowly through the nostrils.

"Sat Chit Ananda" Mantra

Sat means "that which never changes" or "truth is absolute being"; *chit* means "consciousness"; *ananda* means "bliss"—"absolute bliss consciousness."

1. Inhale "sat."
2. Exhale "chit."
3. Inhale "ananda."
4. Exhale the breath slowly through the nostrils.

Meditation

Many of us think the purpose of meditation is to tune out and let go of stress. The latter is certainly a pleasant side effect, but the true purpose of meditation is to tune into yourself and to feel at peace. The purpose is not to escape life for a while, but to interact with yourself and the world around you in a state of kindness and compassion.

Anyone who studies the history of yoga soon learns that the primary goal of early practitioners was to quiet the mind. Meditation is a technique for triggering the relaxation response, allowing the mind to slow down. Practiced meditators report that they experience peacefulness, self-awareness, focus, kindness, and better sleep. A growing body of scientific research suggests that regular meditation may lower blood pressure and reduce anxiety, depression, and insomnia.[3]

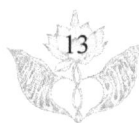

Meditation can be its own practice, or you may integrate it into your yoga practice at any point. B.K.S. Iyengar referred to yoga as "meditation in action," and once said that "yoga is meditation; meditation is yoga."[4]

Grounding Your Meditation Practice

1. Find a comfortable, peaceful place. If you are new to meditation, you might set a timer or an alarm clock for three to five minutes.
2. Position your body:
    a. Chair: Prop a bolster or block, if needed, vertically, from the sacrum, along your spine, and sit so that your feet are on the floor, ankles vertically aligned with the knees. Roll your shoulders back and down, keeping your chin parallel to the floor. Place your hands gently in your lap, palms up or down.
    b. Mat: Sit (on a bolster or blanket if needed), your back erect, your legs cross-legged (with a block under each knee if needed). If your body needs more support, lean against a wall, with or without a bolster or block propped vertically from the sacrum, along your spine. Roll your shoulders back and down, keeping your chin parallel to the floor. (If your body needs to recline, you may lie on your back with a bolster or blanket under the knees and a folded blanket or towel under your head and neck.)
3. Pay attention to the breath, its movement in and out of your lungs and nostrils. Just observe; do not try to control or manipulate the breath.
4. When your mind wanders (and it will!), smile and return to the breath. You may use a mudra (pp. 11–12) or a mantra (pp. 12–13) to help you focus the breath. Let go of self-judgment. Do not try to stop your thoughts or empty your mind. Just notice and anticipate the next breath.
5. At the end of your practice, if you are on the floor, slowly roll to one side and press up to a seated position; if you are in a chair, stay in alignment.
6. Bring your hands to Anjali Mudra (p. 11), bow your head, and say aloud or silently, "Namaste," to give grace and gratitude.
7. Thank your body, mind, and soul for all its good efforts.

Meditation is simple but not always easy. Distraction and frustration are a natural part of the process, even for seasoned meditators, but sticking with it brings remarkable benefits. Practice, practice, practice. Experiment with meditating at different times of day: first thing in the morning, mid-afternoon, just before bed. Once you find a time that works for you, aim to practice at that time every day, even if only for two or five minutes. You can meditate unguided, incorporating a mudra (pp. 11–12) or a mantra (pp. 12–13), or guided, with your favorite meditation audio or video[5] or a script (pp. 15–18), which you may wish to record so that you can close your eyes and sink into the sound of your own voice. The key to a successful, fulfilling meditation practice is finding the right fit for you.

"Sa Ta Na Ma" Meditation

This meditation improves brain function and reportedly prevents or slows down Alzheimer's disease.[6] *Sa* means "birth"; *ta* means "life"; *na* means "death"; *ma* means "rebirth"—affirming the eternal phases of being.

1. Inhale "sa" while touching the tip of the thumb to the index finger.
2. Exhale "ta" while touching the tip of the thumb to the middle finger.
3. Inhale "na" while touching the tip of the thumb to the ring finger.
4. Exhale "ma" while touching the tip of the thumb to the pinky finger.

Do this meditation anytime, anywhere, to relieve stress and induce calm; and, for a deeper practice, work your way to this eleven-minute round:

1. Repeat the mantra aloud for two minutes.
2. Repeat the mantra in a whisper for two minutes.
3. Repeat the mantra silently for three minutes, moving your tongue but making no sound.
4. Repeat the mantra in a whisper for two minutes.
5. Repeat the mantra aloud for two minutes.
6. Inhale slowly through the nostrils, raising your arms in the air at least to chest level, shaking your arms and fingers and, if possible and pleasurable, your whole body and spine.
7. Exhale slowly through the nostrils.
8. Repeat the round once or twice if you want to move and release more energy in your body.

"So Hum" Meditation

So hum means "I am that"; "that" refers to the universal consciousness, one's chosen divine being, the goodness within—affirming "I am universal consciousness," "I am light within," and "I am filled with goodness."

1. Inhale through the nostrils for a slow count of four.
2. Exhale through the nostrils for a slow count of four.
3. At the back of your throat, still breathing through the nostrils, create a soft sound of "so" on the inhalations and a soft "hum" on the exhalations.
4. Count the beats for each "so" and each "hum," like a metronome in your mind, then even out the length of your inhalations and exhalations by gently expanding whichever is shorter.
5. Continue for two to three minutes, then come back to your normal breath.

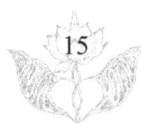

Ho'oponopono, a Hawaiian Prayer Meditation

Ho'o means "to make"; *pono* means "right," so its repetition means "doubly right," that is, being right with both self and others. What empowers this process is your emotion and the universe's inspiration to forgive and to love—so try this meditation if you have hurt someone. Breathe evenly, steadily, while you say these phrases quietly aloud or silently in your mind:

1. Inhale "I'm sorry." (repentance)
2. Exhale "Please forgive me." (forgiveness)
3. Inhale "Thank you." (gratitude)
4. Exhale "I love you." (love)
5. Repeat the pattern for three rounds or until you feel more lightness in your body.

Peaceful Loving Meditation

This meditation[7] sets a powerful intention—for the day if practiced in the morning, for an event if practiced beforehand, for anytime!

1. Focus on this thought: "I am a peaceful soul; my aim today is to radiate peace to every person I encounter."
2. As other thoughts emerge, let go of judgment, and silently say the following sequence:
   - I am a peaceful soul.
   - I am a peaceful, loving soul.
   - My mind is filled with peace.
   - I radiate peace to the world.
   - I feel the gentle waves of peace flowing across my mind.
   - As these peaceful thoughts emerge in my mind, I feel the stillness, and silence embraces my mind.
   - I am a peaceful soul.
   - I am a peaceful, loving soul.
   - My mind feels light and free from worries.
   - I realize my true nature is peace.
   - Peaceful thoughts flow through the mind, and I feel myself becoming light.
   - I am a being of light, shining like a star.
   - I radiate peace and light to the world.
   - Light and peace radiate within me, and waves of peace and light shine like a lighthouse.
   - I allow my heart to shine with peace.
   - I am a peaceful, loving soul.
3. Repeat until you can experience the stillness of mind that comes when your soul is at peace.

Loving-Kindness (Metta) Meditation

This meditation's phrases[8] are designed to evoke a feeling of compassion toward yourself and others. Over time, you'll find it possible to focus on the feeling, allowing the words to fade.

1. Breathe naturally, focusing on the breath going in and out, in and out.
2. Place your attention on the middle of your chest, around your heart.
3. Repeat silently, feeling the resonance of the words: "Love, love, love, may my heart be filled with love."
4. To help access the feeling of loving-kindness, you might imagine any person or animal that inspires your caring (e.g., gazing at a baby's face, stroking a kitten's soft fur).
5. Experience this feeling of warmth and love, the sense of healing and soothing, through your whole body. Let it wash over and through you as you repeat silently:
   - May I be well, healthy, and strong.
   - May I be happy.
   - May I abide in peace.

   This stage can be challenging. Spend some days or weeks cultivating loving-kindness for yourself before you move on (in the next step) to sending that feeling to others.
6. Bring to mind someone you like and respect. Send them these feelings of warmth and caring as you repeat silently:
   - May you be happy. (This is sufficient if you prefer a simpler script.)
   - May you be well.
   - May you abide in peace.
7. Bring to mind another person you like and respect. Send them this feeling of loving-kindness as you repeat silently:
   - May you be happy.
   - May you be well.
   - May you abide in peace.
8. Bring to mind someone you barely know, about whom you feel neutral (e.g., a passerby on the sidewalk, a fellow passenger on the bus, an acquaintance you pass in the corridor at work). Send them these feelings of warmth and caring as you repeat silently:
   - May you be happy.
   - May you be well.
   - May you abide in peace.

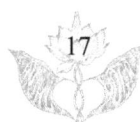

   The feeling of loving-kindness may understandably weaken when you focus on people with whom you're only peripherally connected. If this happens, simply return to an earlier step to rekindle the feeling.
9. Bring to mind someone with whom you recently became irritated or upset (e.g., a slow driver on the way to work this morning, a coworker who blew off a team meeting last week, not someone who has hurt you deeply). Send them these feelings of warmth and caring as you repeat silently:
   - May you be happy.
   - May you be well.
   - May you abide in peace.

10. If you wish, and if you are able to do so at this early stage in your practice, bring to mind someone who has hurt you in the past, toward whom you carry bitterness, hatred, or resentment. Including such a person in your practice does not mean you condone or approve of what they've done; you're lovingly allowing yourself to release some pain and anger. Send them this feeling of loving-kindness as you repeat silently:
    - May you be happy.
    - May you be well.
    - May you abide in peace.
11. Radiate warmth and love to everyone in your town or city, your state, the nation, the world, repeating silently:
    - May you all be happy.
    - May you all be well.
    - May you all abide in peace.
12. Bring your attention back to yourself so the feeling of loving-kindness fills your whole being. Breathe in peacefully; breathe out peacefully. Feel at peace with yourself and with the world.
13. Slowly let the feeling of loving-kindness abate, and return to focusing solely on your breathing.

There's no right or wrong way to practice meditation: just breathe. Meditation is accessible to everyone, everywhere, at every stage of life. To supplement our teachings, check out YouTube meditation channels, meditation websites, TED talks, podcasts, and apps for your phone or tablet (Calm, Insight Timer, Simple Habit, Headspace, and Breethe). Just making a conscious effort is a monumental step toward inner peace and calmness.

Now that we've learned the internal workings of yoga, let's bring in the physical postures.

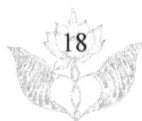

1. B.K.S. Iyengar, *Light on Life: The Yoga Journey to Wholeness, Inner Peace, and Ultimate Freedom* (Emmaus, PA: Rodale Books, 2005), pp. 77–81; "Meditation: In Depth," National Center for Complementary and Integrative Health, last updated April 2016, www.nccih.nih.gov/health/meditation-in-depth; Sara Lazar, "Harvard neuroscientist: Meditation not only reduces stress, here's how it changes your brain," posted May 26, 2015, https://hms.harvard.edu/news/harvard-neuroscientist-meditation-not-only-reduces-stress-heres-how-changes-your-brain; Victor Dubin, "Low Pressure Tactics: Using Yoga to Lower Blood Pressure," *Yoga for Healthy Aging*, posted November 26, 2019, https://www.yogauonline.com/yoga-for-heart-disease/low-pressure-tactics-using-yoga-lower-blood-pressure.

2. Thich Nhat Hanh, *Being Peace* (Berkeley, CA: Parallax Press, 2005), p. 15.

3. See #1.

4. B.K.S. Iyengar, "The Path of Yoga." Interview by Margot Kitchen, July 5, 1990. *The Newsletter*, Spring 1991, Iyengar Associations of Greater New York and Massachusetts.

5. Our favorites are Richard Miller's yoga nidra and Sharon Salzberg, Joseph Goldstein, and Jack Kornfield's metta meditation, all searchable on YouTube.

6. Alissa Sauer, "How Meditation Can Slow Alzheimer's," posted June 20, 2016, https://www.alzheimers.net/2013-11-25-how-meditation-can-slow-alzheimers.

7. Author unknown.

8. Multiple online sources provide scripts for Loving-Kindness (Metta) Meditation.

Yoga facilitates living your authentic wisdom.
~Linda Anastasia Ransom

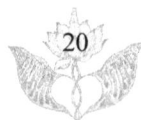

CHAPTER III

Heating Up: Flowing Asanas

One of the most important components of Healing Chair Yoga is that you listen to your body and practice *ahimsa* (kindness, non-harming), which includes not pushing yourself too far too fast. We are not here—in this world, on the mat, in the chair—to change who we are; we are here to meet ourselves where we are.

In this chapter, you will learn postures (asanas) that open the feet; the wrists, hands, and fingers; the shoulders and neck; the heart; and the hips; that twist the spine to relieve tension; and that strengthen physical balance. These asanas are not meant to be done in one yoga session. Pick two or three asanas (more or fewer per your body's guidance) from each of the seven asana sections in this chapter, as well as one restorative asana from the next chapter, to practice daily or at least three times a week (fewer per your body guidance).

As you begin your asana practice, it's essential to remember your alignment (p. 5) and pranayama (Ujjayi suggested, p. 8). Adding mudras (pp. 11–12) and mantras (pp. 12–13) is optional.

Before you begin any posture, be sure to read its entire procedure. These asanas are held in tune with the breath—specifically, as instructed in this book, for three to five breaths. If this measure doesn't work for your body, count the number of times you breathe within thirty seconds, and use that as your timer. Likewise, repeating the asanas per practice session is only a suggestion. Listening to your body is the most important component of yoga.

Foot Openers

Let's start with the feet. These faithful, oft-neglected companions carry us around; they serve as our very foundation and connection to the earth. The feet are a powerful energy source: according to Ayurvedic medicine, they contain *marma* points, gateways to the connective tissue and the *nadis*, subtle lines that channel energy to every cell of the body. The feet (literally) ground our balance system, communicating with our senses and muscles to keep us upright and stable. Every time we kick off our shoes, stretching the toes and arches, flexing the ankles, we're reminded that happy, healthy feet are integral to a happy, healthy body.

Benefits:
- Improve balance and posture, and hence promote confidence
- Strengthen toes, arches, heels, and ankles
- Increase flexibility and mobility
- Improve stability and body awareness when we stand, walk, hike, bike, run

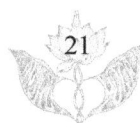

- Enhance circulation
- Relieve foot tightness, aches, and pains (may help prevent plantar fasciitis and arthritis)

Grounding Your Fancy Footwork

1. Seated in a chair, in Tadasana alignment notice your feet. How do you stand? Is your body weight evenly distributed, or is it more on the insides or outsides, on the heels or the balls? Are your toes relaxed?
2. Evenly distribute your weight across both feet.
3. Stretch the toes of both feet wide until you can see daylight between them. (For happy, healthy feet and toes, lift and spread your toes whenever you can.)
4. Hold for three to five breaths and release.
5. Repeat one or two times.

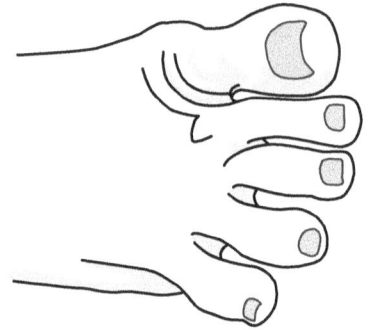

Foot Massage

1. Seated in a chair, in Tadasana alignment, cross your foot over the opposite knee.
2. Use your opposite hand to gently massage the entire foot, from toes to heel.
3. Interlace the fingers with the toes as if you are holding hands with your foot—pinky finger under the base of the little toe, ring finger slid under the base of the next toe, and so on, until your fingers and toes are firmly connected, thumb on top of the big toe.
4. Gently spread your fingers as wide apart as you can.
5. Hold for three to five breaths and release.
6. Repeat one or two times.
7. Do the sequence with the other foot. (Five minutes of this asana alone will help stimulate the connective tissue via *marma* points.)

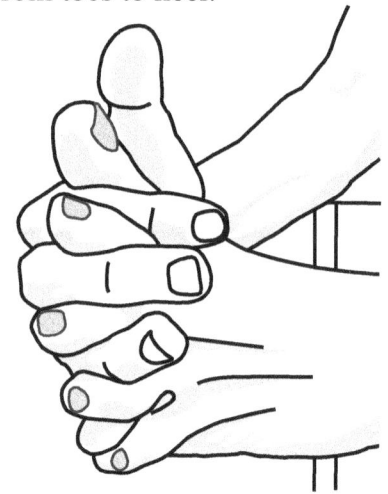

Arch Stretch I

1. Seated in a chair, in Tadasana alignment, cross your foot over the opposite knee, and grasp the toes with the same-side hand.
2. Gently pull your toes back, in a flexed position, until you feel a stretch in the arch of your foot.
3. Hold for three to five breaths and release.
4. Repeat one or two times.
5. Do the sequence with the other foot.

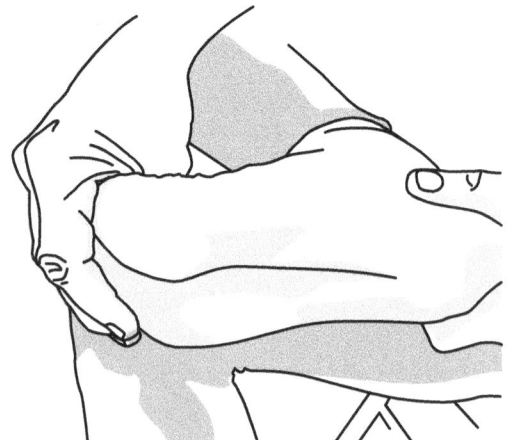

Arch Stretch II

1. Place a towel on the floor in front of your chair.
2. Seated in a chair, in Tadasana alignment, grab the towel with the toes of one foot and, without moving your foot along the floor, pull the towel toward you by scrunching and lengthening your toes. Try to pick up the towel with your toes!
3. Hold for three to five breaths and release.
4. Repeat one or two times.
5. Do the sequence with the other foot.

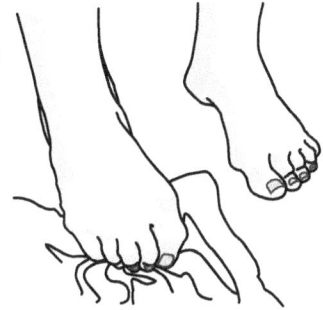

Flex, Point, Floint

1. Seated in a chair, in Tadasana alignment, extend one leg, and flex the foot so that the heel energetically pushes away from the body, and the top of the foot gently pulls up and toward the body. Hold for three to five breaths and release.
2. Unflex the ankle and point the toes out and toward the floor, so that the heel slightly pulls up and into the body. Hold for three to five breaths and release.
3. Leading with the ball of the foot, pull the toes back toward the body as the heel energetically pulls up and into the body (floint: flex + point). Hold for three to five breaths and release.
4. Repeat one or two times.
5. Do the sequence with the other leg.

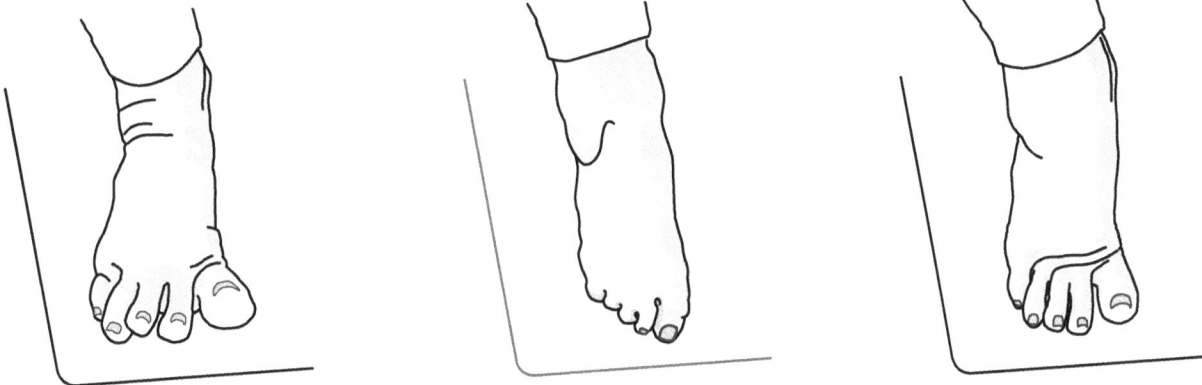

Ankle Rolls

1. Seated in a chair, in Tadasana alignment, extend one leg and gently rotate that foot at the ankle, making circles with the toes, for three to five breaths.
2. Gently rotate that foot in the opposite direction for three to five breaths.

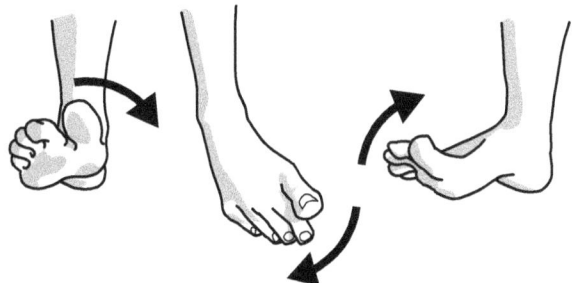

3. Do the sequence with the other foot.
4. Repeat one or two times.

Ball Massage

1. Seated in or standing behind a chair, in Tadasana alignment, evenly distribute your body weight across both feet.
2. Consciously root the sole of each foot at these four points:
    a. the ball of your foot directly under the big toe
    b. the ball of your foot directly under the pinky toe
    c. the inside of the heel
    d. the outside of the heel
3. Gently shifting your weight onto one foot, lift the other foot and place a racquetball or tennis ball underneath. Keep the feet parallel and hip-width apart for balance. (If standing, you may hold on to the chair back to keep your balance.)
4. Gently pressing down on the lifted foot, roll the ball along the entire sole—the arch, the heel, the ball, the inside and outside edges—to warm up your foot and get a feel for the motion and pressure needed to stabilize the ball. It may feel tingly!
5. Shifting your body weight to intensify the pressure on the lifted foot, work the ball along the sole as follows:
    a. Place the ball in the pronounced depression where the toes meet the first and second metatarsals. Allow the toes to relax and perhaps release over the ball. Squeeze, roll, and release. Repeat for thirty to sixty seconds, exploring the sensation, applying more pressure as desired, and breathe.
    b. Roll the ball to the middle of the foot, slightly above the arch. Again, squeeze, roll, and release repeatedly for thirty to sixty seconds.
    c. Shift the ball to the arch, and repeat the process. This position in particular may produce an intense physical response, so just keep breathing and back off if it hurts.
    d. Roll the ball to where the arch meets the heel, and repeat the process.
    e. Place the ball directly under the heel, and repeat the process. To keep the ball from popping out, apply pressure vertically.
6. Redistributing your body weight, roll the ball along the entire sole for a massage.
7. Straighten your leg and settle that foot back on the floor. Notice the differences between the two sides of your body, from your feet all the way up to your shoulders and neck.
8. Do the sequence with the other foot. (Five minutes of this asana alone will help stimulate the connective tissue via marma points.)

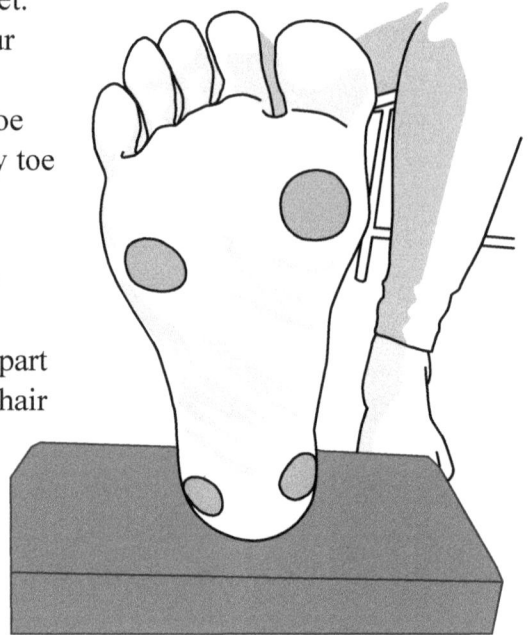

Virabhadrasana I (Warrior I), Flexed Toes at the Wall, with Block

1. Align the short edge of your mat against a wall.
2. Stand facing the wall, a few inches from it, in Tadasana alignment.
3. Place both hands on the wall, shoulder-width apart, and step one of your legs back into a Warrior I lunge, planting that foot at a 45-degree angle.
4. Square your hips to the wall.
5. Flex the toes of your front foot, and place them up against the wall, spreading the toes as wide as you can.
6. Place a block between the wall and the knee of your front leg, and press the block into the wall.
7. Hold for three to five breaths.
8. Do the sequence with the other foot.
9. Repeat one or two times.

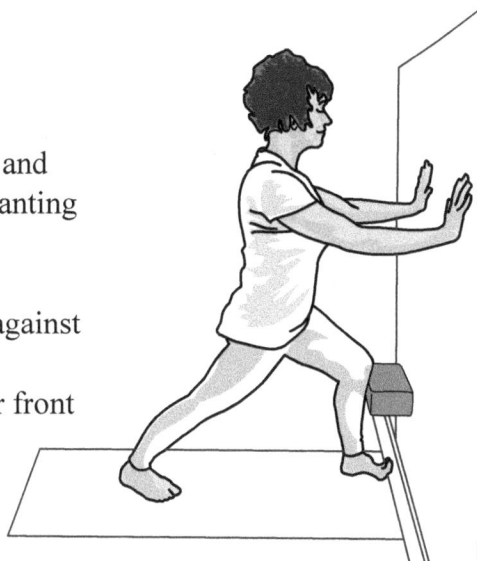

Toes on Block, Heel Up and Down

1. Align the short edge of your mat against a wall, and place a block—largest surface flat, short end aligned with the wall—about six inches from the wall.
2. Stand a few inches behind the block, facing the wall, in Tadasana alignment.
3. Place both hands on the wall, shoulder-width apart, and press the ball of one foot on the block such that the arch aligns with the edge of the block.
4. Slowly raise the heel of that foot, inhaling, then lower it, exhaling, until you feel a good stretch. Do this for three to five breaths.
5. Do the sequence with the other foot.
6. Repeat one or two times.

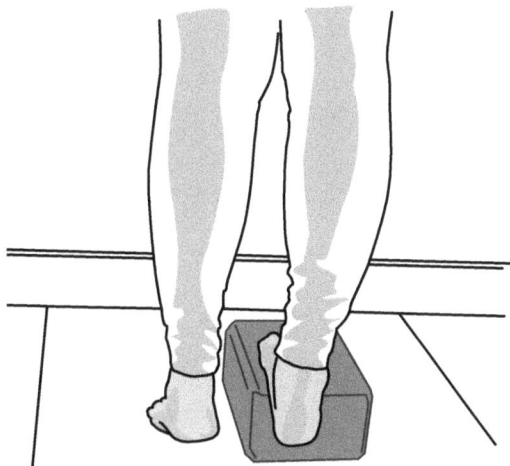

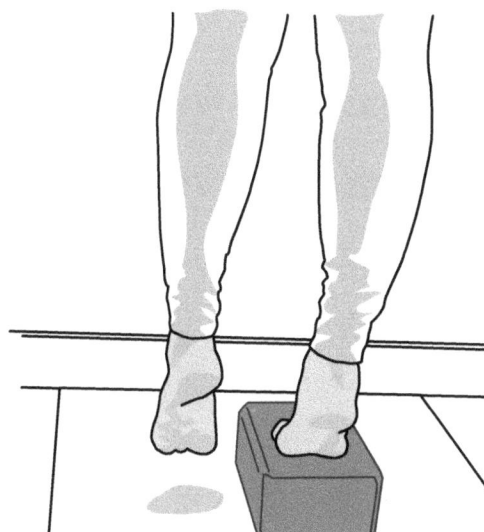

Virabhadrasana I (Warrior I), Back Heel Up and Down

1. Align the short edge of your mat against a wall.
2. Stand facing the wall, a few inches from it, in Tadasana alignment.
3. Place both hands on the wall, shoulder-width apart, hips squared to the wall.
4. Step back with one foot, toes pointing forward in a variation of Warrior I, keeping your feet hip-width apart and your hips squared.
5. Slowly raise and lower the back heel for three to five breaths. Feel the strength of the back leg as the ball of the front foot stays anchored to the mat.
7. Do the sequence with the other foot.
8. Repeat one or two times.

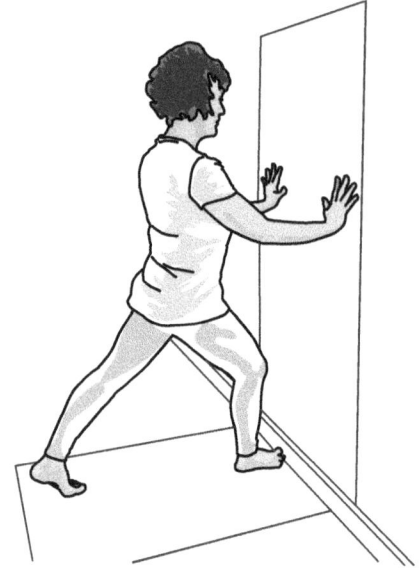

Wrist, Hand, and Finger Openers

How would we function in today's world if we didn't have hands? Our hands operate the computer, cell phone, remote control, steering wheel, and the list goes on. Repetitive movements can create weakness and stiffness in our wrists, hands, and fingers. Texting Thumb, Smartphone Thumb, Gamer's Thumb—these are real diagnoses of a condition known as *de Quervain's tenosynovitis*, pain in the tendons on the thumb-side of the wrist. Before the digital revolution, it was known as Mommy Thumb, from the frequent picking-up and holding of a newborn. Simple exercises performed daily can strengthen the wrists and keep the hands and fingers flexible well into our later years.

Benefits:
- Relieve pain and swelling
- Reduce joint damage
- Strengthen and stretch the muscles in the hands and forearms
- Strengthen the muscles around the joints for better support
- Increase blood circulation to the hands, warming the muscles and joints
- Increase the circulation of synovial (joint) fluid
- Regain mobility and flexibility
- Improve range of motion

Shake, Shake, Shake

1. Seated in a chair, in Tadasana alignment, gently shake out your hands for three to five breaths.
2. Pause for one breath.
3. Repeat one or two times.

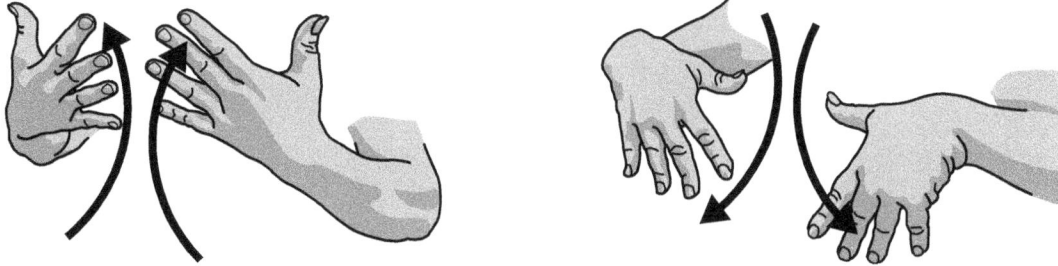

Spread Fingers Wide and Make a Ball

1. Seated in a chair, in Tadasana alignment, spread the fingers of both hands as wide as you can, palms up, keeping your elbows close to the body.
2. Hold for three to five breaths and release.
3. Squeeze the fingers into a tight ball.
4. Hold for three to five breaths and release.
5. Gently shake out your hands.
6. Repeat one or two times.

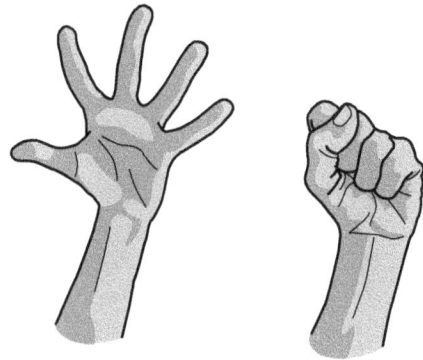

Wrist Circle and Shake

1. Seated in a chair, in Tadasana alignment, make fists with both hands, palms down, keeping your elbows close to the body.
2. Rotate your wrists in a circular motion, first clockwise simultaneously, then counterclockwise, for three to five breaths in each direction.
3. Gently shake out your hands.
4. Repeat one or two times.

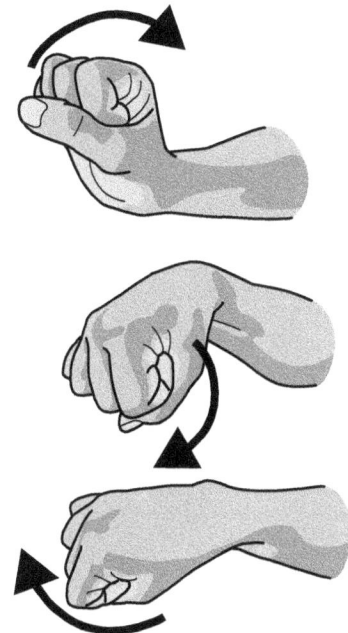

Stop-Sign Hands

1. Seated in a chair, in Tadasana alignment, extend one of your arms in front of you, and make a Stop gesture with that hand, palm facing forward, fingers pointing toward the ceiling.
2. With your other hand, gently pull your fingers back while the heel of the extended hand presses forward.
3. Hold for three to five breaths and release.
4. Gently shake out your hands.
5. Do the sequence with the other arm.
6. Repeat one or two times.

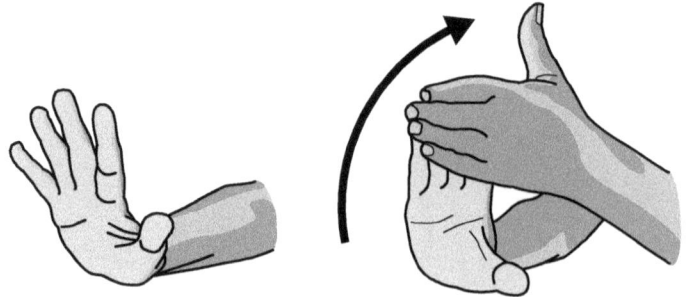

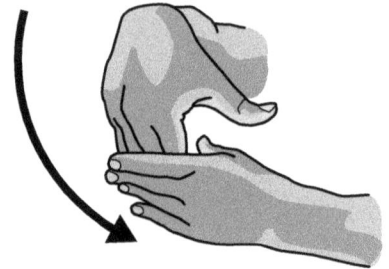

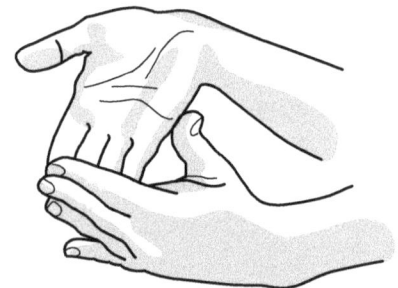

Reverse Stop-Sign Hands

1. Seated in a chair, in Tadasana alignment, extend one of your arms in front of you, palm down.
2. With your other hand, gently press your fingers down toward the floor, then toward your body while your wrist presses forward.
3. Hold for three to five breaths and release.
4. Gently shake out your hands.
5. Do the sequence with the other arm.
6. Repeat one or two times.

Palm Up

1. Seated in a chair, in Tadasana alignment, extend one of your arms in front of you, palm up.
2. With your other hand, gently press your fingers down toward the floor, then toward your body while your wrist presses forward.
3. Hold for three to five breaths and release.
4. Gently shake out your hands.
5. Do the sequence with the other arm.
6. Repeat one or two times.

Karate-Kid Hands Sprinkling Fairy Dust

1. Seated in a chair, in Tadasana alignment, extend both arms in front of you.
2. Point all your fingers (including the thumbs) toward the floor, and gently press them toward your elbows.
3. Bring the thumbs and pointer fingers together to make the Karate-Kid crane-beak shape.
4. Pressing up through the tops of your wrists, raise your arms overhead as high as you can toward the ceiling.
5. Hold for three to five breaths.
6. Slowly return your hands to your knees, gesturing with your fingers as if sprinkling fairy dust.
7. Gently shake out your hands.
8. Repeat one or two times.

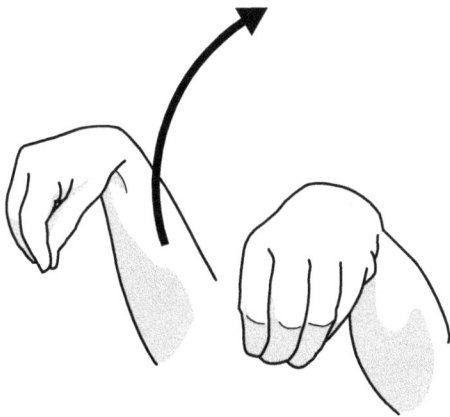

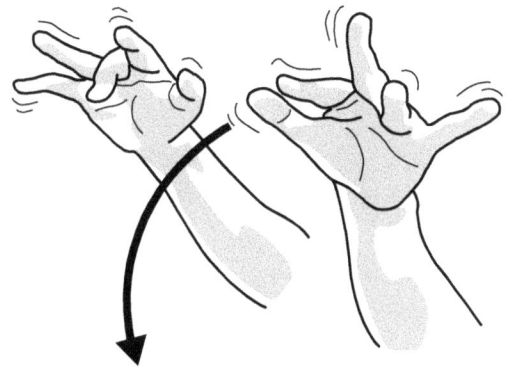

Tennis-Ball Squeeze

1. Seated in a chair, in Tadasana alignment, place a tennis ball (or racquet ball) in the palm of your hand.
2. Squeeze for three to five breaths and release.
3. Do the sequence with the other hand.
4. Gently shake out your hands.
5. Repeat one or two times.

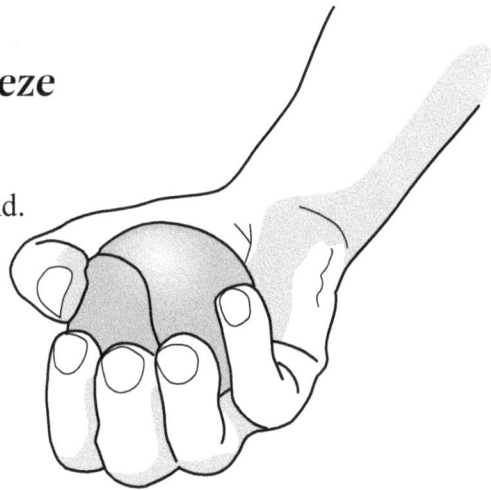

Fist Flexion

1. Seated in a chair, in Tadasana alignment, rest your forearms on your thighs, hands at the knees, palms up.
2. Make fists with both hands, firm as if holding a pencil, and raise them toward your body, bending only at the wrists.
3. Hold for three to five breaths and release.

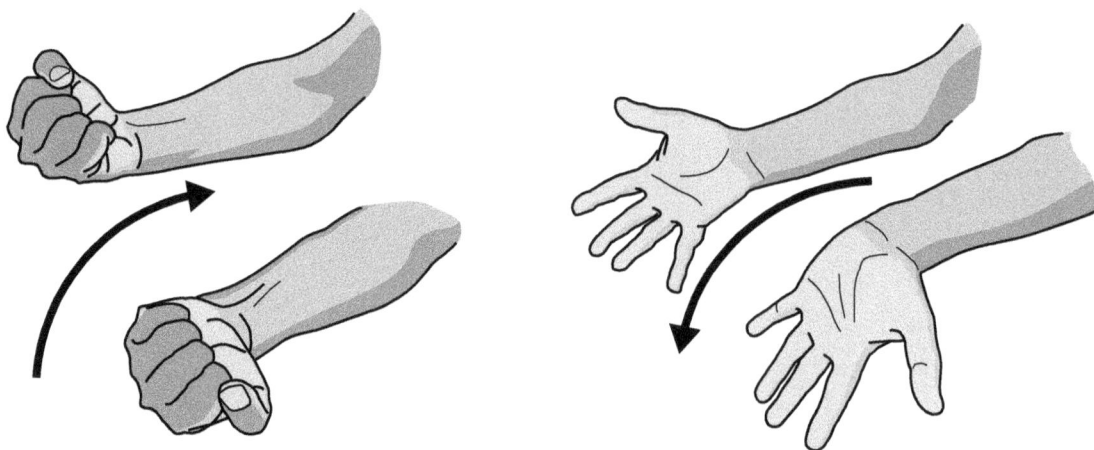

4. As you lower your fists to your knees, slowly spread your fingers wide.
5. Gently shake out your hands.
6. Repeat one or two times.

Thumb Flexion and Extension

1. Seated in a chair, in Tadasana alignment, keeping your elbows close to your body, extend both arms in front of you, palms up.
2. Spread your fingers wide, thumbs stretching outward.
3. Reach your thumbs across the palms, touching the base of the pinky fingers if you can.
4. Hold for three to five breaths.
5. Return your thumbs to the starting position, spreading your fingers wide.
6. Hold for three to five breaths.
7. Gently shake out your hands.
8. Repeat one or two times.

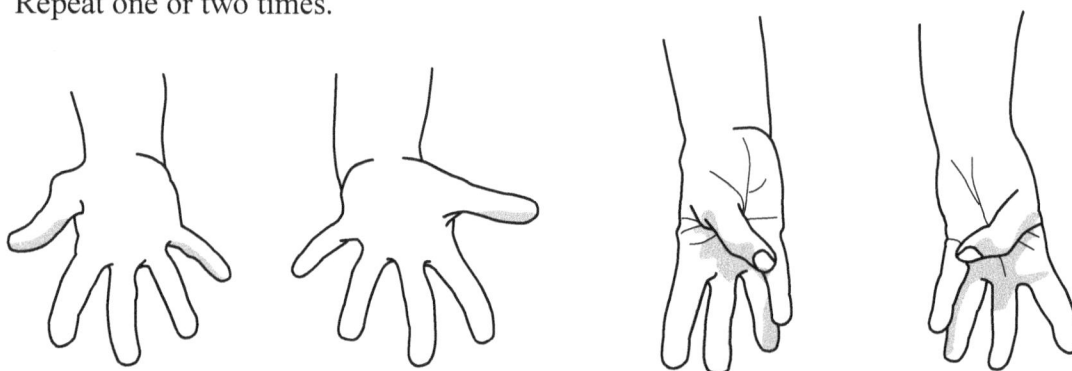

Thumb Pull

1. Seated in a chair, in Tadasana alignment, make a fist with one of your hands, pointing the thumb in a thumbs-up position.
2. Generate resistance with your thumb and hand muscles to keep the thumb from moving.
3. With the fingers of your other hand, gently pull back on your thumb.

4. Hold for three to five breaths and release.
5. Do the sequence with the other hand.
6. Gently shake out your hands.
7. Repeat one or two times.

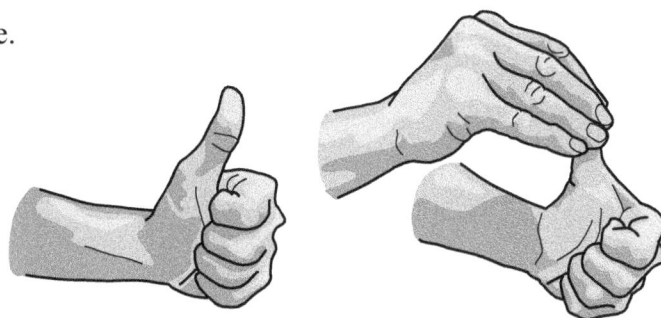

Figure Eights

1. Seated in a chair, in Tadasana alignment, interlace your fingers in a clasped-prayer position at waist height, keeping your elbows close to your body.
2. Move your hands in a figure-eight motion, rotating the wrists completely so that each hand is alternately on top of the other.
3. Continue for three to five breaths.
4. Release the clasp, and gently shake out your hands.
5. Repeat #1–4 one or two times.
6. Raise your arms overhead, and interlace your fingers in a clasped-prayer position.
7. Keeping your fingers interlaced, turn your palms toward the ceiling, straightening your arms as much as your shoulders will allow.
8. Hold for three to five breaths and release.
9. Gently shake out your hands.
10. Repeat #6–8 one or two times.

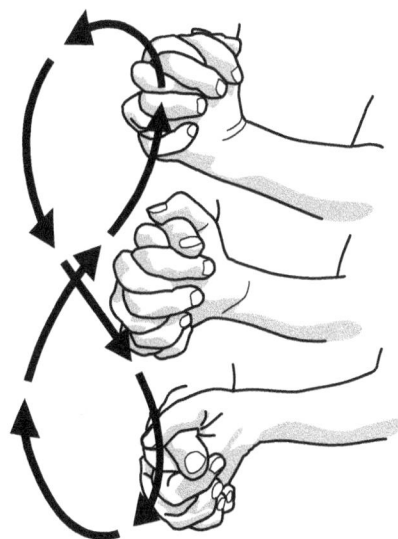

Namaste Hands

1. Seated in a chair, in Tadasana alignment, bring your palms together in front of your face, with your arms touching from wrists to elbows, or as aligned as is possible.
2. Keeping your palms pressed together, slowly spread your elbows apart while lowering your hands to waist height.
3. Stop when your hands arrive in front of your belly button or as soon as you feel a stretch in your wrists.
4. Hold for three to five breaths.
5. Keeping your palms pressed together, slowly raise your hands to face height until your elbows meet.
6. Repeat one or two times.
7. Gently shake out your hands.

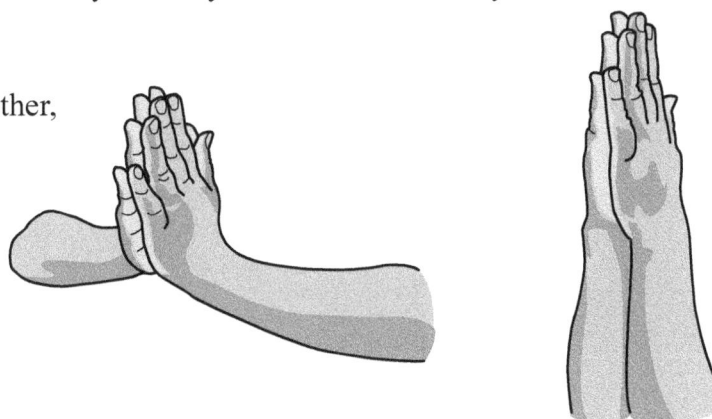

Shoulder and Neck Openers

Rare is the adult who doesn't have a cranky neck, back, or shoulder. Whether caused by injury or by habitually hunching over a computer, cellphone, or steering wheel, rounded shoulders and tight chest muscles are the norm for many of us. Chronic tension or pain then layers deeper and deeper, in the muscles and tendons, restricting our capacity to breathe fully.

Our language is peppered with shoulder idioms relating to struggle, difficulty, or heavy responsibility: shoulder the load, shoulder the burden, have broad shoulders, keep one's shoulder to the wheel, a chip on one's shoulder, a weight off one's shoulders, carry the weight of the world on one's shoulders—even the mythological Atlas was condemned to hold the weight of the heavens on his shoulders. For both physical and emotional stress, our shoulders are a convenient storage place.

Shoulder work is foundational to nearly all Hatha yoga poses. Right now, roll your shoulders up toward your ears, and gently drop them down your back. Is your chest, your heart center, more open? Does your breathing come more easily, and deepen?

Be mindful as you do this work. The shoulder joint is the most mobile joint in the human body. Its large range of motion makes it especially unstable, more prone to injury and dislocation than other, less mobile joints.

Benefits:
- Release tension in the neck, shoulders, chest, and upper back
- Open the trapezius and the scalene muscles of the neck.
- Loosen the scapulae from the network of muscles and ligaments that attach them to the neck and upper spine
- Increase mobility and flexibility
- Improve strength and endurance for the shoulders, neck, and spine
- Foster the natural curvature of the spine

Shoulder and Wrist Warm-Up

1. Seated in a chair, in Tadasana alignment, lift your right hand straight in front of you, palm down. Make a gentle fist, and bend your elbow.
2. Roll the wrist clockwise for three to five breaths, then counterclockwise for three to five breaths. Allow the elbow and shoulder to be part of this movement.
3. Repeat one or two times.
4. Gently shake out your wrist, elbow, and shoulder.
5. Do the sequence with your left hand.

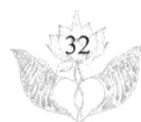

6. Roll both wrists, elbows, and shoulders simultaneously, first in inward circles, then in outward circles, for three to five breaths in each direction.
7. Repeat #6 one or two times.
8. Gently shake out your wrists, elbows, and shoulders.

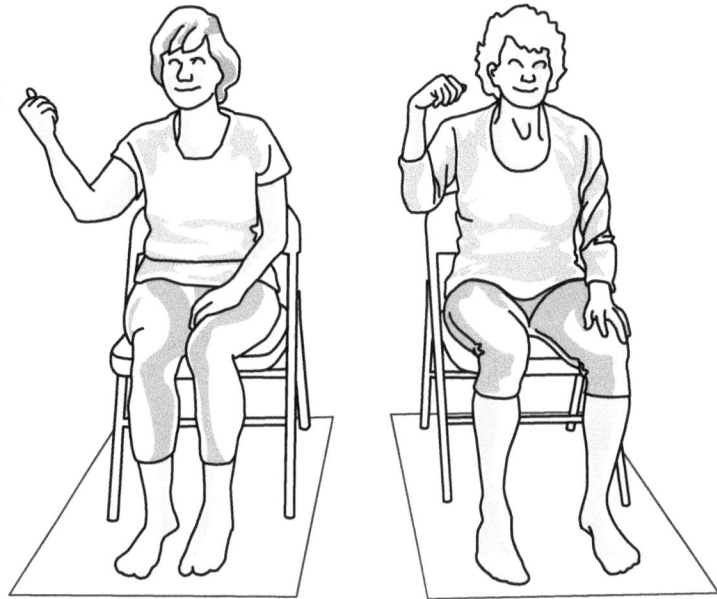

Elbow-Slide Neck Stretch

1. Seated in a chair, in Tadasana alignment, bring your hands to Anjali Mudra (p. 11).
2. Lightly press the palms together. The elbows will slightly lift.
3. Inhaling, slide the palms to the right, across the chest. Allow your neck to follow your hands, unless you have neck strain, in which case, keep looking straight ahead. Hold for three to five breaths, exhaling back to center on the last breath.
4. Inhaling, slide the palms to the left, either following with your neck or looking straight ahead. Hold for three to five breaths, exhaling back to center on the last breath.
5. Repeat one or two times.
6. Gently shake out your hands and arms.
7. Variation: If you have lower-back pain, insert a block lengthwise between your thighs.

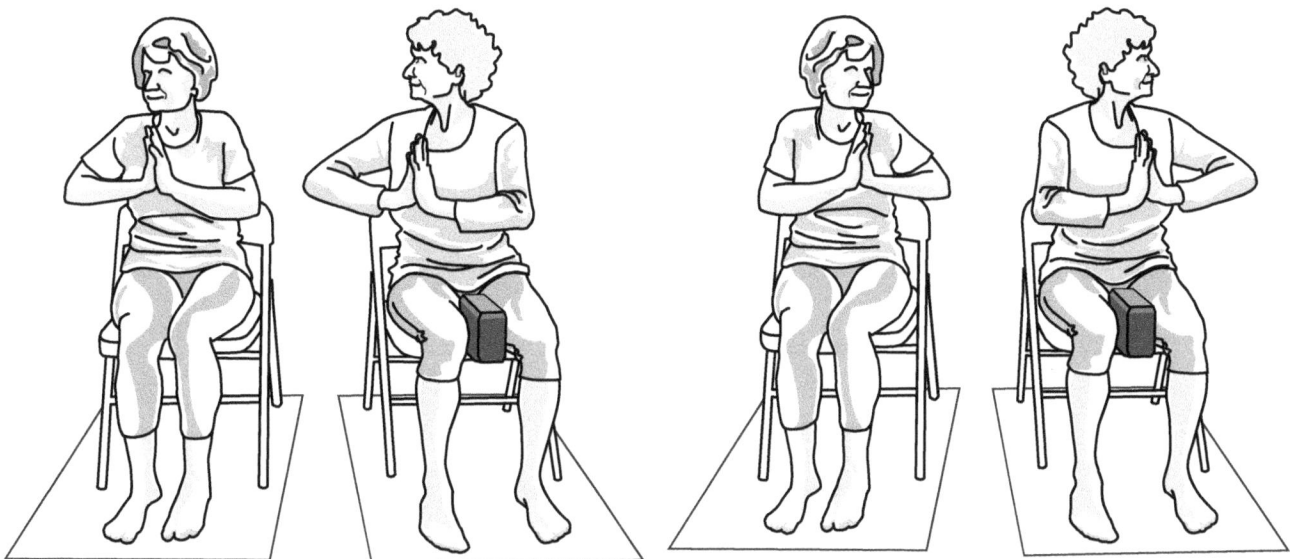

Shoulder Circles

1. Seated in a chair, in Tadasana alignment, fold your arms across the chest, and lightly clasp the inside of the opposite elbows.
2. With your folded arms as one unit, make clockwise circles in front of your body, engaging the shoulder, for three to five breaths. Increase the radius as it feels comfortable.
3. Do the sequence in the counterclockwise direction.
4. Gently shake out your arms.
5. Repeat one or two times.

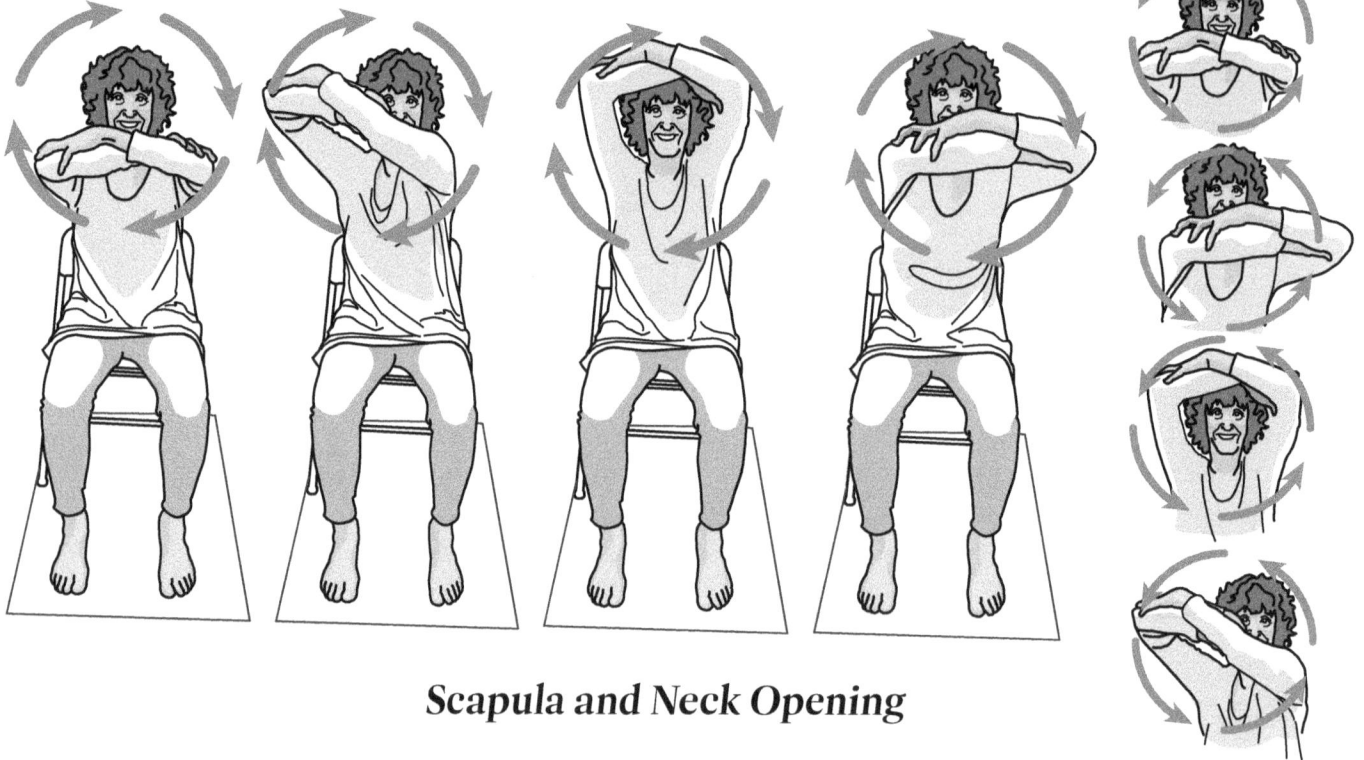

Scapula and Neck Opening

1. Seated in a chair, in Tadasana alignment, extend your arms forward, parallel to the floor.
2. Bend your elbows and place your fingertips on your shoulders.

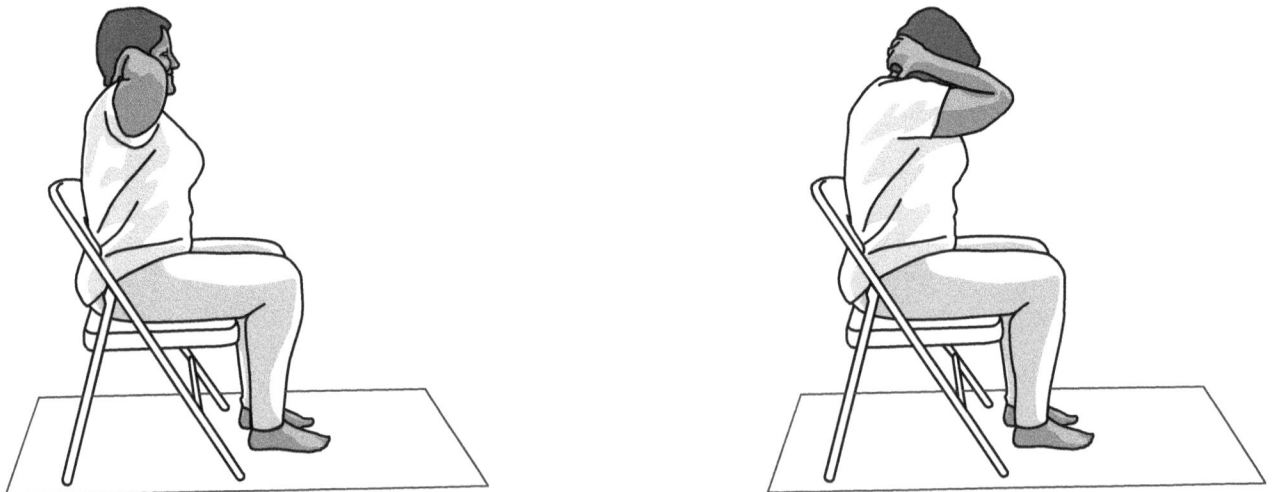

3. Inhaling, draw your elbows out to the sides, pressing the shoulder blades together. You may bow your head forward if your neck feels no pain or strain.
4. Exhaling, draw the elbows forward and together, feeling the shoulder blades slide apart.
5. Repeat #3–4 for three to five breaths.
6. Gently shake out your hands and arms.
7. Repeat one or two times.

Trapezius and Neck Stretch

1. Seated in a chair, in Tadasana alignment, reach both arms behind you, bend your elbows, and clasp the elbows (or as close as you can) with opposite hands.
2. Release your left hand, and place it on the left thigh, with the right hand holding the left arm just above the inside of the elbow (or as close as your body allows).
3. Inhaling, lift the crown of your head toward the ceiling, lengthening the neck.
4. Exhaling, lower the left ear down toward the left shoulder, without moving the shoulder to meet the ear.
5. Drop the right shoulder and breathe into the right side of the neck.
6. Hold for three to five breaths.

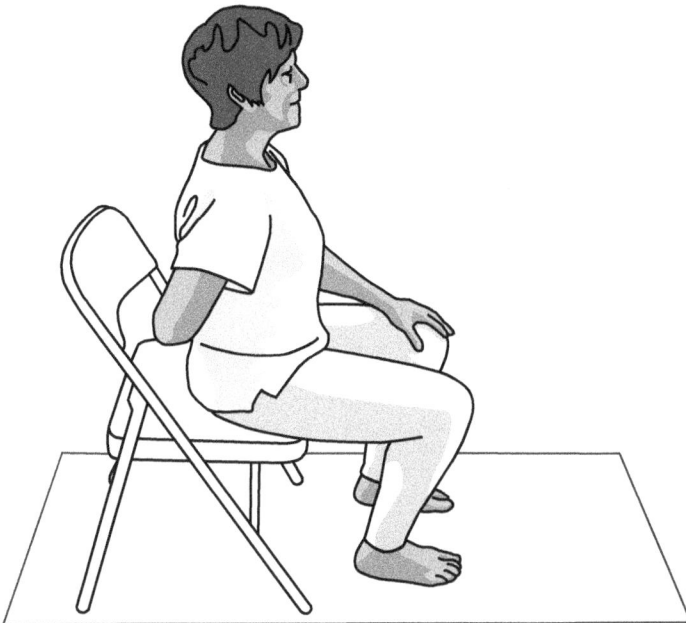

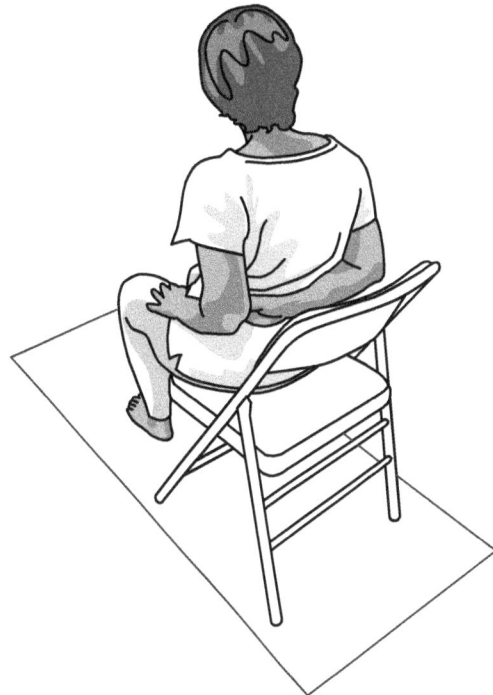

7. Exhaling, release both arms, and bring your head back to center.
8. Do the sequence on the other side.
9. Gently shake out your hands and arms.
10. Repeat one or two times.

Earlobe Tug and Neck Stretch

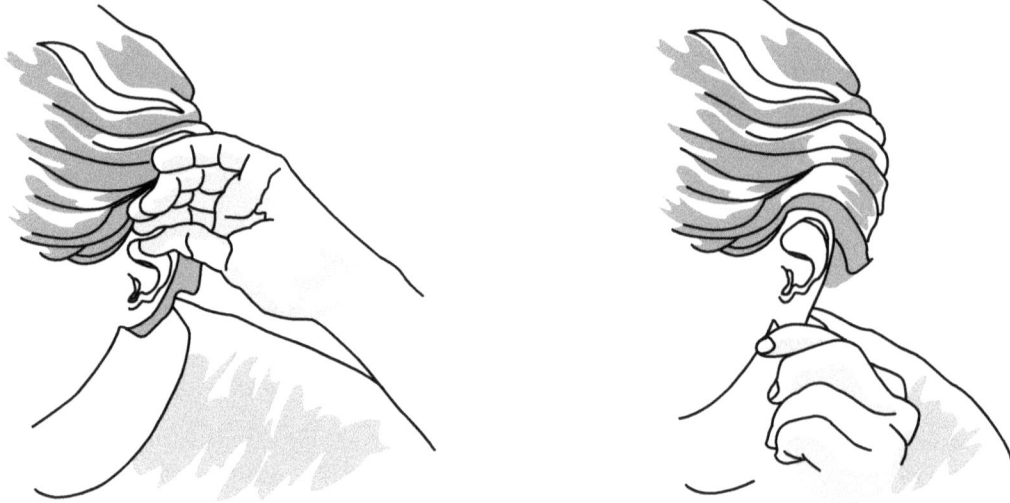

1. Seated in a chair, in Tadasana alignment, lower the right ear to the right shoulder, without moving either shoulder. Notice any tension in the left side of your neck. Bring your head back to center.
2. With the fingers of the left hand, gently massage the left ear, beginning with the top folds for three to five breaths, moving to the middle folds for three to five breaths, then moving to the lobe for three to five breaths, and concluding with three gentle, sustained tugs of the lobe.
3. Lower the right ear to the right shoulder, and notice any changes, perhaps a release of tension in the left side of your neck.
4. Do the sequence with the left ear.

Shoulder Stretch

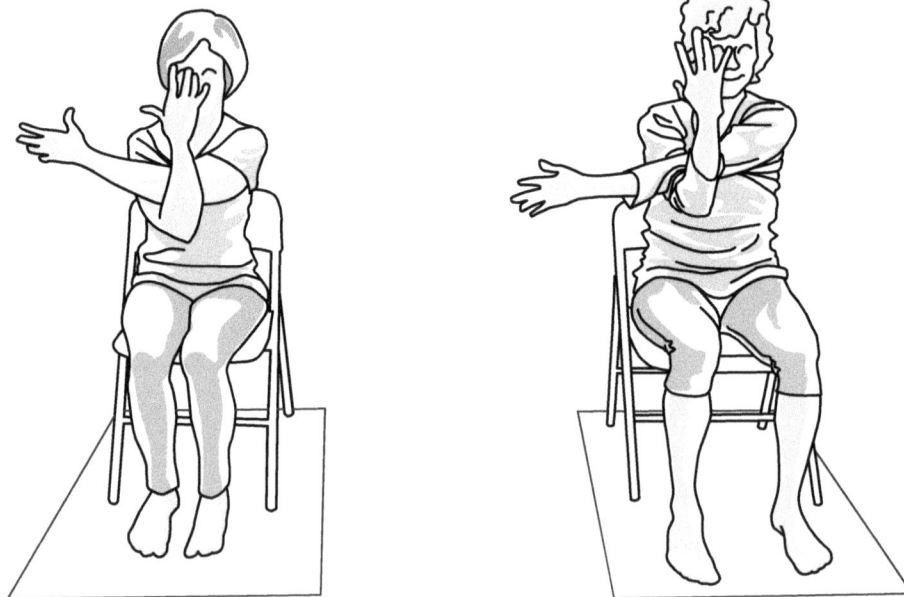

1. Seated in a chair, in Tadasana alignment, extend the right arm across the chest, at collarbone level.
2. Extend the left arm straight in front of you, and rest the right arm in the crook of the left elbow.
3. Bend the left arm up at a 90-degree angle, and gently pull the right arm closer to the body while reaching it farther to the left.
4. Hold for three to five breaths.
5. Do the sequence on the other side.
6. Gently shake out your hands and arms.
7. Repeat one or two times.

Garudasana (Eagle Arms)

1. Seated in a chair, in Tadasana alignment, cross your right arm underneath the left arm, aligning the elbows, and bend the elbows until your hands align, fingers pointing toward the ceiling.
2. Place your right fingers into your left palm, pressing your two hands together. If your hands can't quite touch like that yet, press the backs of the hands together or simply place the right palm on the left shoulder and the left palm on the right shoulder.
3. Gently lift the elbows, reaching the fingertips toward the ceiling if they are not on the shoulders.

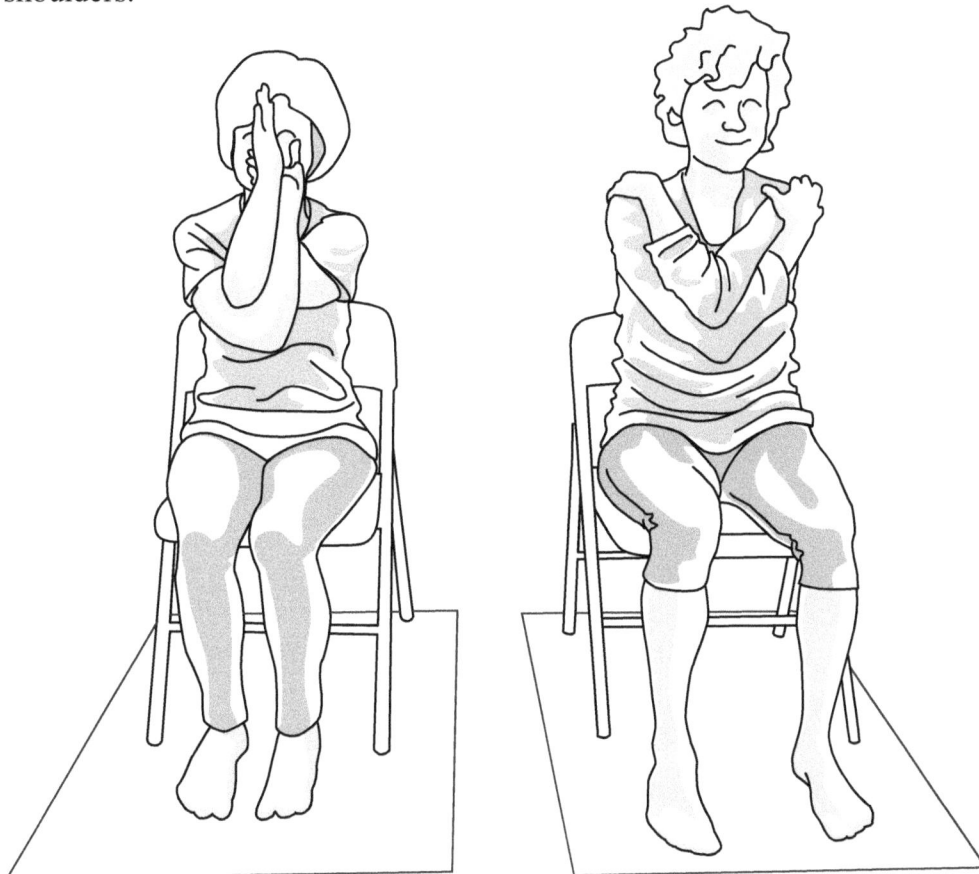

4. Hold for three to five breaths, focusing on the inhalations and exhalations, and keeping your gaze fixed and soft.
5. Unwind your arms and shake them out gently.
6. Do the sequence on the other side, left arm underneath right arm.
7. Repeat one or two times.

Gomukhasana (Cow Face)

1. Seated slightly forward in a chair, in Tadasana alignment, extend the left arm straight in front of you, palm facing left.
2. Gently swing that arm around behind your back, bend the elbow, and place the back of hand on your low back.
3. Scoot that hand up the spine, resting it comfortably between the lower rib cage and the shoulder blades.
4. With your right hand, dangle a yoga strap over the right shoulder, palm facing inward.
5. Find the strap with your left hand, and "walk" your hands toward each other, along the strap, keeping your elbow aligned vertically over the shoulder, until you feel a safe, adequate stretch.
6. Hold for three to five breaths.
7. Release the strap at one end, relax your arms at your sides, and shake them out gently.
8. Do the sequence with the right arm.
9. Repeat one or two times.

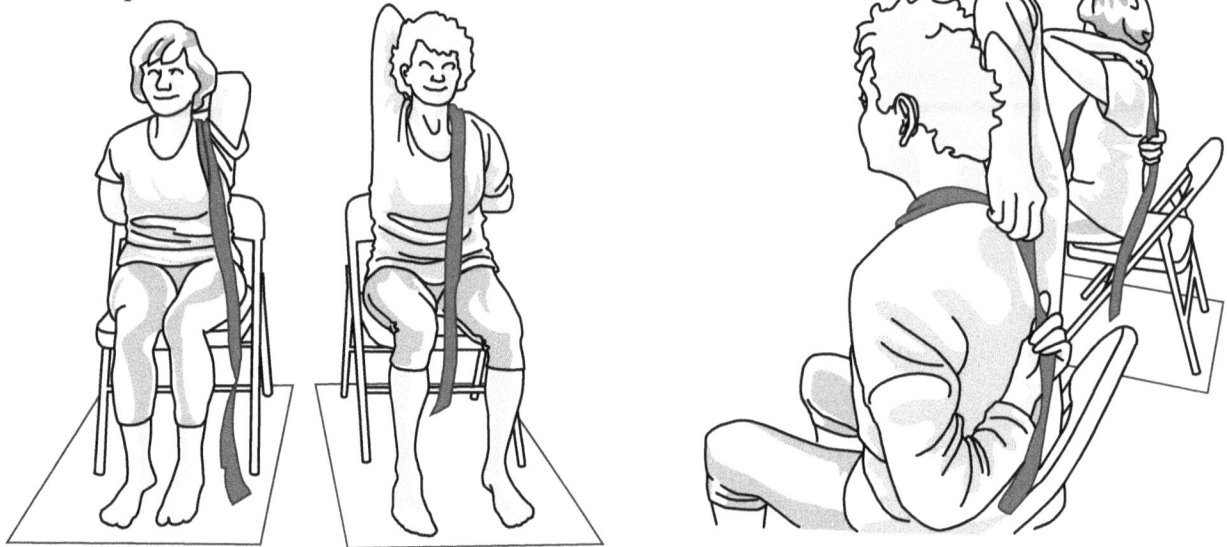

Shoulder Opening with Strap

1. Seated slightly forward in a chair or standing, in Tadasana alignment, tautly clasp a yoga strap shoulder-width between your hands, arms extended straight in front of you. If your shoulders feel strained or pinched, widen your hold on the strap.
2. Slowly raise the arms overhead, incrementally widening your hold on the strap to provide

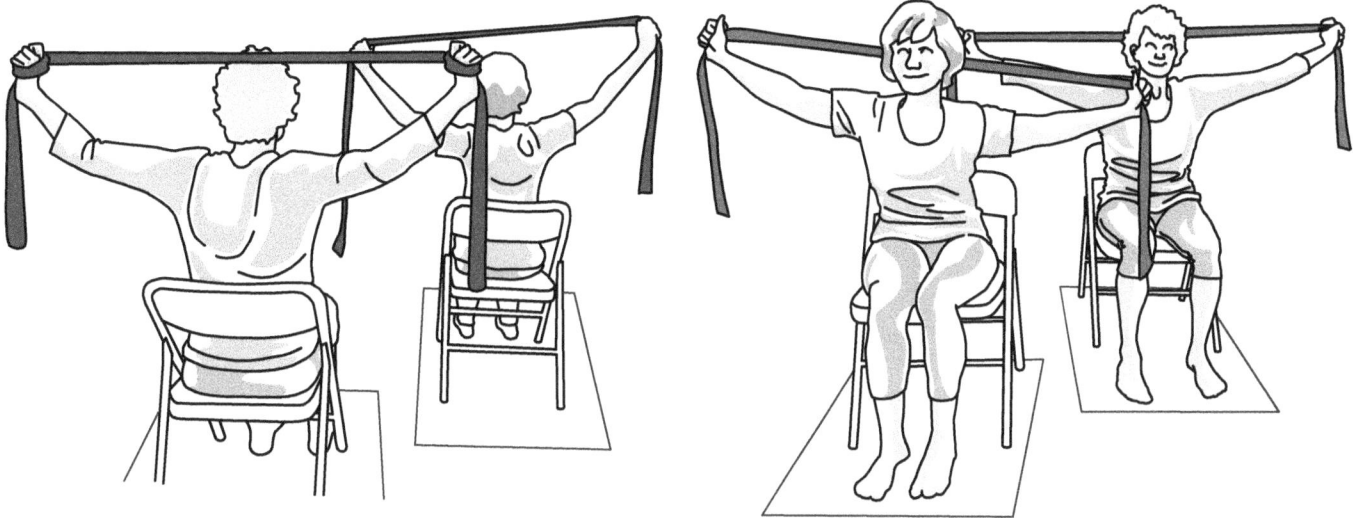

unrestricted movement for the shoulders. Keep the back-body firm, the core engaged, the rib cage stable, and the torso and head facing forward.

3. Inhaling, slowly lower the strap to shoulder height. Hold for three to five breaths.
4. On the last exhale, raise the strap back overhead, maintaining a smooth, continuous movement of the arms.
5. Repeat #3–4 one or two times.
6. With the strap overhead, further widen your hold on it.
7. Inhaling, lower the strap down the back-body, incrementally widening your hold so as not to strain or pinch the shoulders. Hold for three to five breaths.
8. On the last exhale, raise the strap back overhead, maintaining a smooth, continuous movement of the arms.
9. Repeat #7–8 one or two times.
10. Release the strap and notice the sensation in your shoulders. Repeat the sequence one or two times.

Adho Mukha Svanasana (Downward-Facing Dog) at the Wall

1. Align the short edge of your mat against a wall.
2. Stand facing the wall, about one foot away, in Tadasana alignment.
3. Place your hands on the wall, shoulder-width apart, at shoulder level, index fingers pointing up so that the wrist creases form a horizontal line.
4. Keeping the above alignment in the hands and shoulders, step back until your arms and torso are parallel to the floor, hips stacked over the feet.

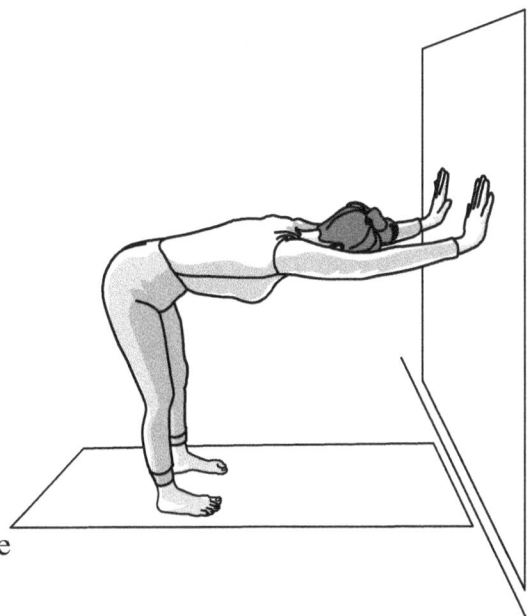

5. Firmly connect to the wall with both hands, and use the energy from this contact to help elongate the spine as you press the hips away from the wall.
6. Engage the core and the shoulders as you keep lengthening the spine, knees slightly bent. Your ears should be aligned with your elbows.
7. Hold for three to five breaths.
8. Walk your feet toward the wall, stopping about one foot away, and come back to Tadasana alignment.
9. Repeat one or two times.

Clock at the Wall

1. Align the short edge of your mat against a wall.
2. Stand in Tadasana alignment, with your right side to the wall, about one foot away, left arm loose at your side.
3. Extend the right arm straight overhead, in the 12 o'clock position, palm facing the wall. Hold for three to five breaths.
4. Without bending the elbow, and keeping the core engaged, slowly move your hand backward, from 12 o'clock to 1, maintaining the forward-facing position of the rib cage to keep the hips squared. Hold for three to five breaths.
5. Without bending the elbow, slowly move your hand from 1 o'clock to 2, and perhaps to 3 o'clock, holding for three to five breaths at each increment. If you feel any tingling in the arm, lessen the rotation backward or step farther from the wall for a wider rotation; if you feel pain, stop.

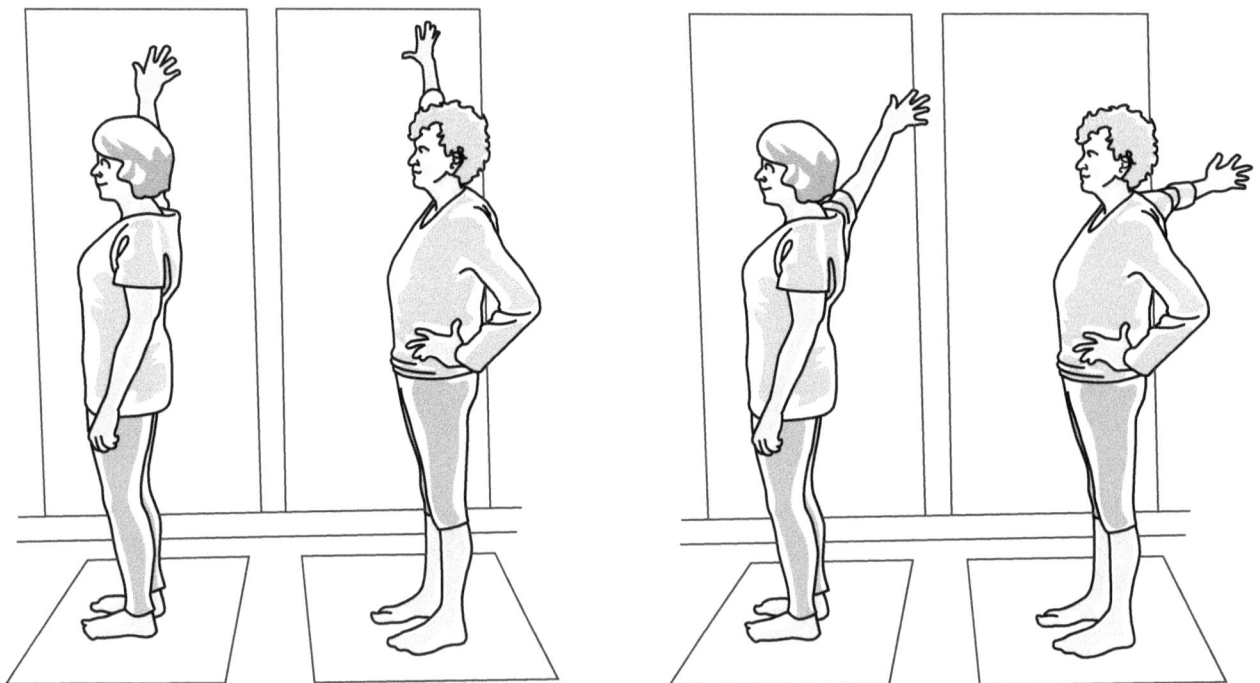

6. You should feel a stretch in the front right shoulder or down the right arm; to intensify the stretch, move closer to the wall.
7. Do the sequence with your left side to the wall, moving the left arm to the 11, 10, and perhaps 9 o'clock positions, holding for three to five breaths at each increment.

Heart Openers

Are you a desk-sitter by day, a couch potato by night? Do you have lower back pain, a heavy heart? Heart openers, also known as gentle backbends, activate the heart chakra, the "seat of the soul." Leading from the center of your chest allows you to tap into your feelings, gaining emotional clarity and control. Lifting the chest, moving the shoulders back, and lengthening the front and back of the body stretches the body all over and physically increases your energy.

Benefits:
- Decrease isolation, depression, and anxiety by (symbolically) expanding compassion and connection with others
- Break through and release stress
- Help tone the spine
- Increase the lungs' breathing capacity, which opens the mind and heart to new possibilities
- Promote feelings of trust by stretching the abdominal muscles and internal organs
- Relieve tightness and pain in the back and shoulders
- Increase blood circulation
- Stimulate the thyroid, pineal, and pituitary glands

Grounding Heart Meditation

1. Sit in a chair, in Tadasana alignment, feet parallel and hip-width apart on the floor.
2. Close your eyes, and bring your hands to Anjali Mudra (p. 11).
3. Inhaling, silently ask, "What makes me grateful?" Exhaling, you may conjure a person, a significant event, or something small, like finding the perfect parking space today. What comes to mind is exactly what needs to.
4. Inhaling, eyes still closed, bring love and thankfulness into your heart.
5. Exhaling, extend your arms to the sides, straight out from the shoulders, palms facing the ceiling. You may feel tingling energy in your hands as you focus on the intention to share love and gratitude with everyone you encounter today.
6. Slowly raise the arms to the goalpost position or fully overhead.
7. Hold for three to five breaths.
8. Draw your hands into prayer position and down the midline of your body. Feel the energy and mindfulness of this heartfelt love.
9. Inhale, keeping your hands in Anjali Mudra; and exhale, bringing your hands straight out to the sides, palms up.

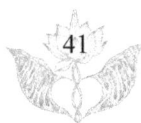

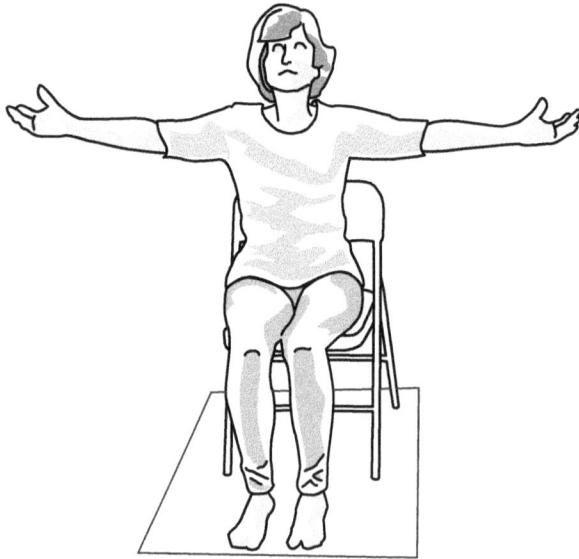

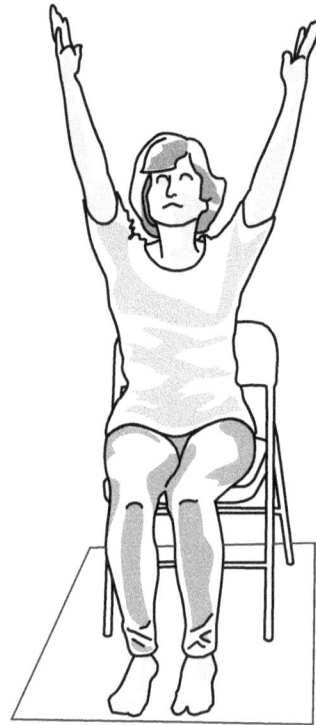

10. Inhale, raising the arms to the goalpost position or fully overhead, looking up slightly, keeping the neck long.
11. Exhale, drawing your hands back to prayer pose at heart center.
12. Repeat #4–9 one or two times, noticing the warmth created in your heart.
13. Close by recommitting to your intention to share loving-kindness with everyone you encounter today, by sending a kind smile, thought, or gesture.

Cat-Cow Flow

1. Sit in a chair, in Tadasana alignment, hands on the knees, and inhale fully.
2. Exhaling, round your back like a mad cat, from lower to upper back, sliding your hands to the front of the knees to deepen the stretch, looking inward, at your heart center. Hold for three to five breaths.
3. Inhaling, lift your head and heart, gently arching your back like a cow's spine, keeping the neck long, landing your gaze toward where the wall and ceiling meet. Hold for three to five breaths.
4. Repeat the sequence one or two times.

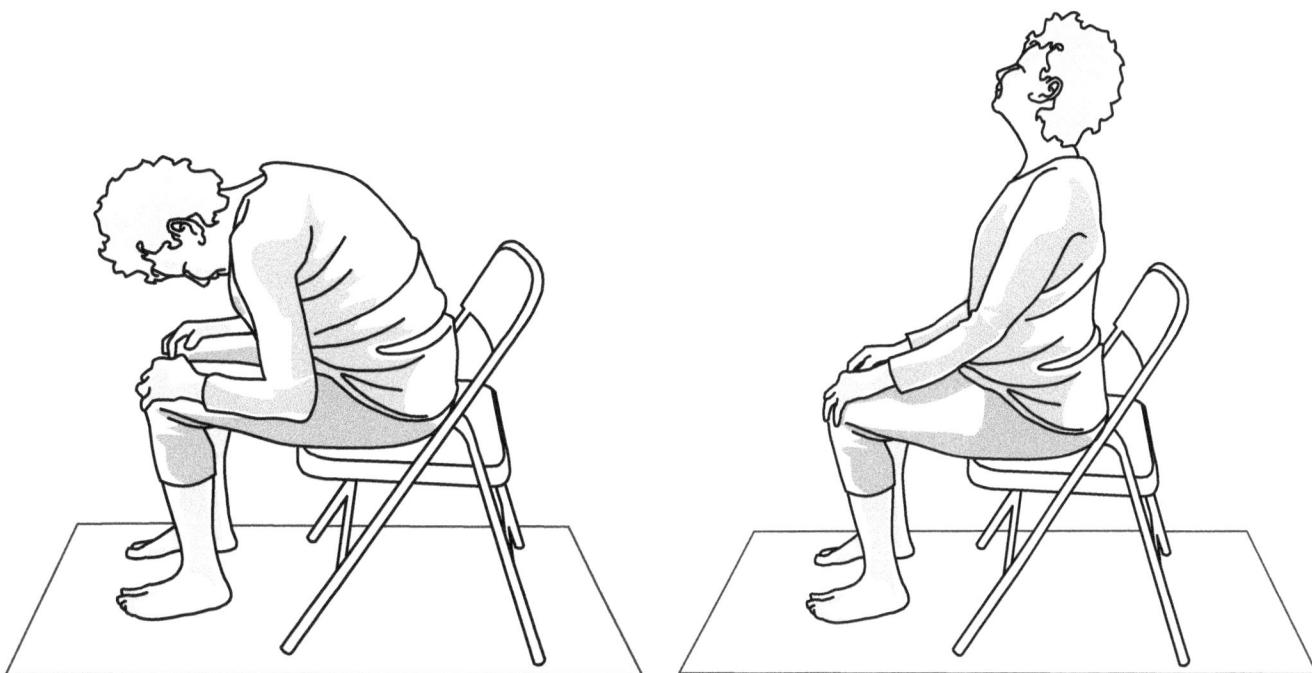

Salamba Setu Banda Sarvangasana (Bridge)

1. Lying on a mat, bend your knees, planting the feet, and reach your fingertips toward the heels, grazing them if your body allows.
2. On an inhale, slowly lift your hips toward the ceiling, rolling up the spine, from lower to upper back, keeping your feet and arms in contact with the mat, and broadening the collarbones as you draw your heart center upward, too.
3. Hold for three to five breaths.
4. On an exhale, slowly lower the hips to the floor, rolling down from upper to lower back.
5. Repeat one or two times.

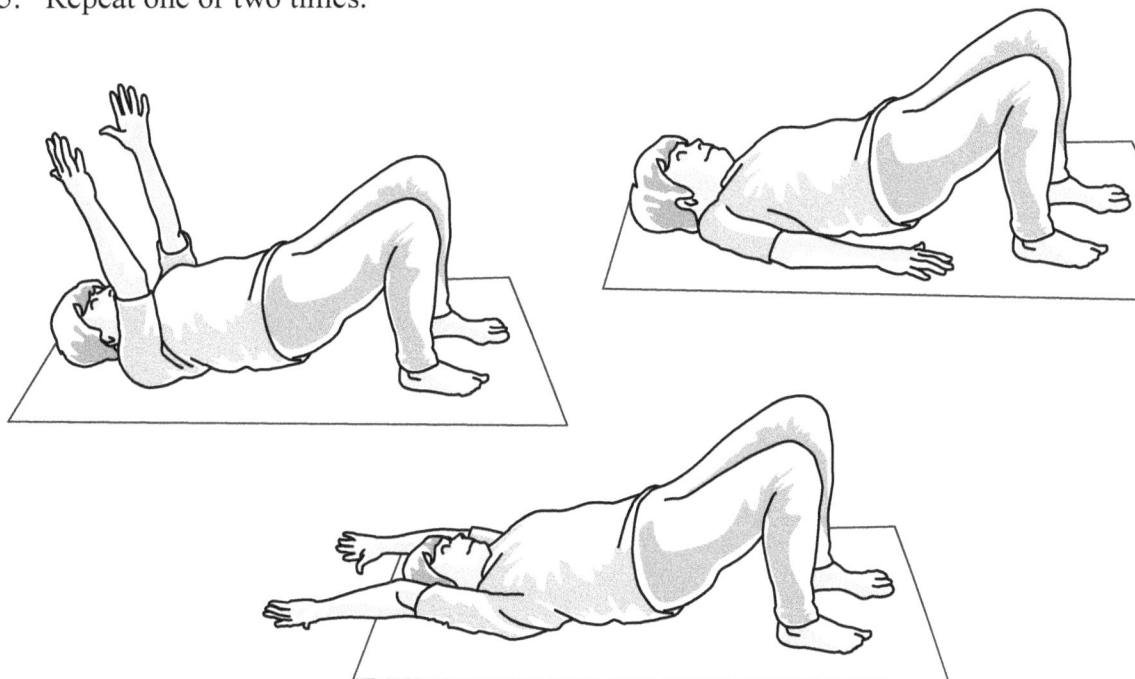

6. Variation: Flowing Bridge: As you lift your hips in #3, reach your arms, palms facing each other, to the ceiling and draw them overhead, elbows toward the ears. Pause. On the exhale, move your hands back toward the ceiling and down to your hips, rolling down through the spine, hips touching the floor at the same time as your arms.

Adho Mukha Svanasana (Downward-Facing Dog) to Urdhva Mukha Svanasana (Upward-Facing Dog)

1. Stand facing the seat of a chair, about two feet away, in Tadasana alignment.
2. Inhaling, bend your knees and engage your core as in Tadasana alignment. Extend your arms to bow forward and hold the sides of the chair.
3. Exhaling, step back approximately another foot. Draw your hips back so that the ankles are vertically aligned with the knees and hips, and the elbows are aligned with the ears. Hold for three to five breaths. Feel the depth of the stretch. This is called Healing Chair Yoga Downward-Facing Dog.
4. Inhaling, come forward into a plank. The wrists, elbows, and shoulders are vertically aligned but not locked.

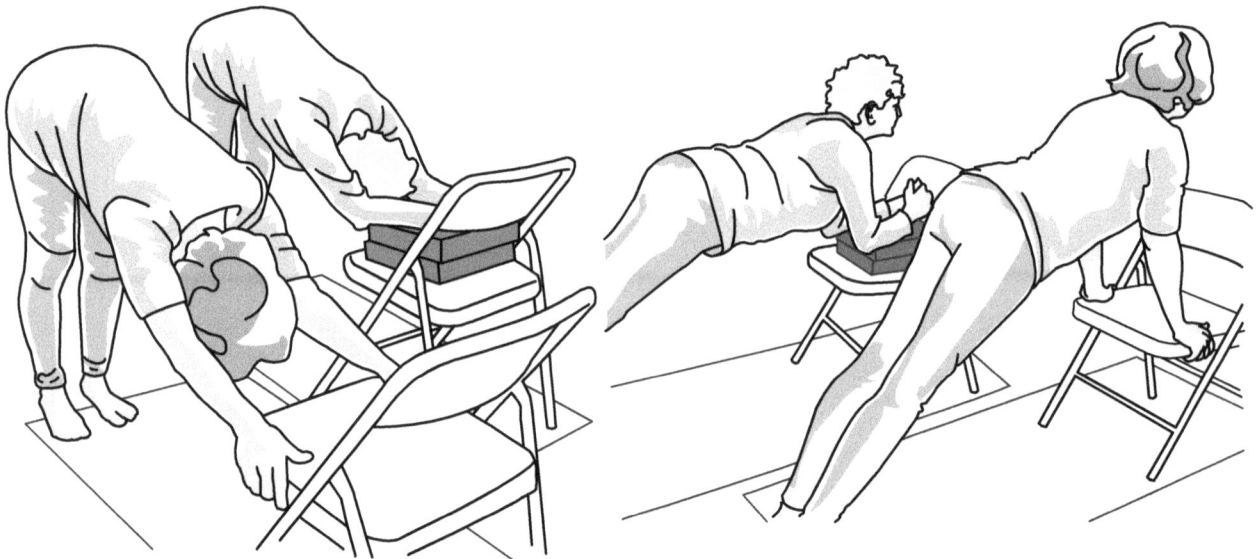

5. Exhaling, lengthen your mid-sternum away from the heels and toward the back of the chair, keeping the lift in your lower belly. Hold for three to five breaths. This is called Healing Chair Yoga Upward-Facing Dog.
6. Repeat this flow one or two times.
7. Variation: If Downward-Facing Dog and Upward-Facing Dog put too much weight on your wrists, modify both poses by coming down to your elbows, either on the seat of the chair or on a block (if you need a higher surface).

Virabhadrasana I (Warrior I)

1. Place a bolster, pillow, or rolled blanket in front of a chair, with the long side up against the chair's front legs.
2. Sit sideways in the chair, in Tadasana alignment, facing right, feet parallel and hip-width apart on the floor.
3. Keeping the right foot planted, place your left knee on the bolster to come into a lunge. Both legs ideally should be bent at a 90-degree angle, right knee directly over right ankle, left hip directly over left knee.
4. Keeping your alignment, bring your hands to Anjali Mudra (p. 11), and gaze toward where the wall and ceiling meet. Keep the neck long and the shoulders back and down, away from the ears. If it is comfortable for your shoulders, raise your arms to a goalpost position or fully overhead.
5. Hold this posture, moving in and out of various arm positions, for three to five breaths.
6. Do the sequence on the left side.
7. Repeat one or two times.

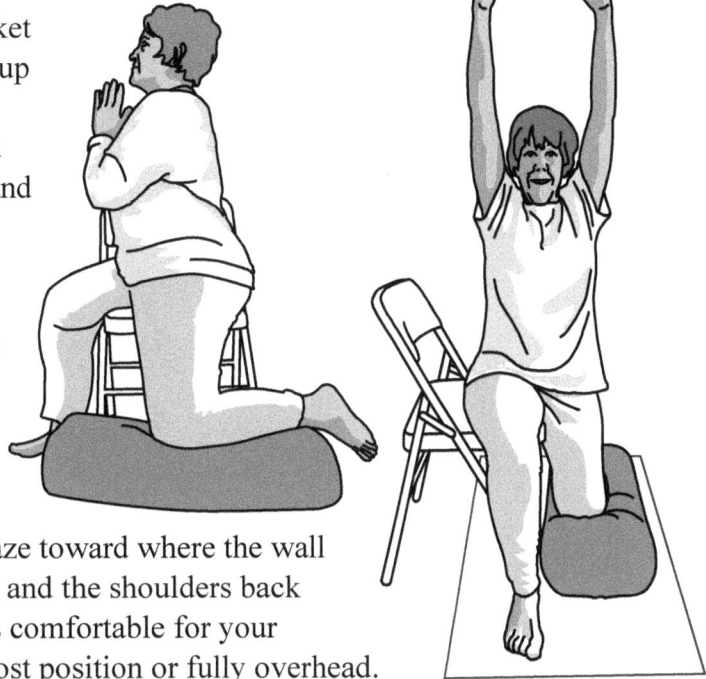

Viparita Virabhadrasana (Reverse Warrior)

1. While holding Warrior I (above), bring the hand of the bolstered knee to the same-side thigh, front, side, or back.
2. Sliding your hand to the lower thigh, gently arch your back, lifting your heart, keeping the neck aligned with the spine, and gaze toward where the wall and ceiling meet.
3. Reach your other arm to the ceiling, palm facing inward, or place that hand on your heart. If the back, neck, or shoulders experience any strain, ease up on the posture.
4. Hold for three to five breaths.
5. Do the sequence on the other side.
6. Repeat one or two times.

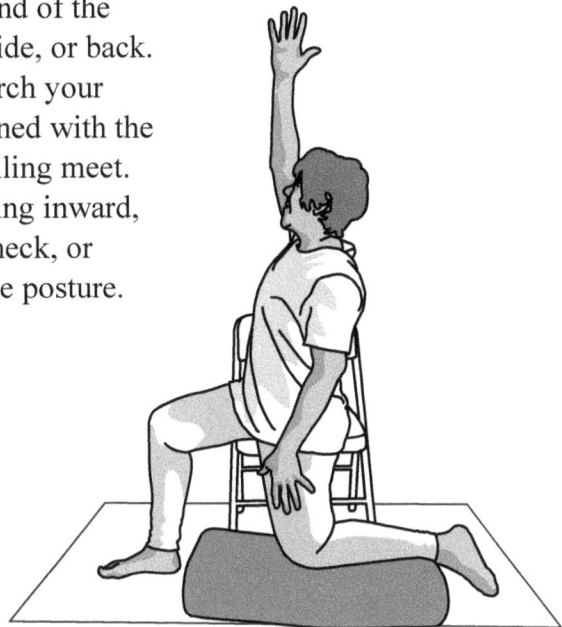

Virabhadrasana I (Warrior I) to
Viparita Virabhadrasana (Reverse Warrior) Flow

1. While holding Warrior I (p. 45), with your hands in Anjali Mudra (p. 11) or your arms in a goalpost position or fully overhead, take three to five breaths.
2. Transition to Reverse Warrior (p. 45). Hold for three to five breaths.
3. Do the sequence on the other side.
4. Repeat this flow one or two times.

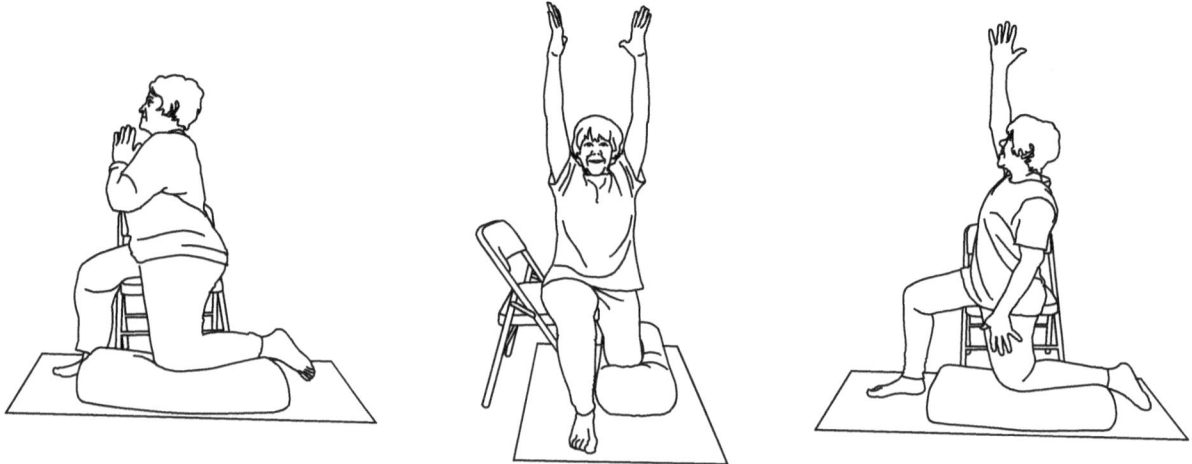

Twists

Stand up straight! Stop slouching! When you were a kid, did your parent or grandparent, even a teacher, chide you about your poor posture? When we sit or stand for long periods of time, our spine tends to slump, compressing the vertebrae and draining us of energy. Twists lengthen the spine, creating space between the vertebrae, facilitating energy flow. As you physically "wring out" your body, your brain and spirit may feel cleansed and purified as well!

Benefits:
- Restore and retain the spine's natural range of motion by rotating the spine and stretching the muscles of the back
- Compress and massage the organs of the abdomen, including the digestive organs
- Stimulate digestion and metabolism
- Flush toxins from the body more efficiently
- Push stagnant blood from, and resupply blood to, the kidneys, liver, and spleen
- Calm the nervous system and quiet the mind

Doing Twists Safely

If you have a back injury, chronic back pain, or degenerative disk disease, please approach these asanas with caution, and practice them only with an experienced yoga teacher. To prevent a back injury, consciously coordinate the breath and your movement as follows:

1. As you inhale, lengthen the spine, leading with the head and neck.
2. As you exhale, twist from the lower spine, working up the spine sequentially through the vertebrae, turning the neck last.

Vakrasana (Twist) Seated

1. Seated in a chair, in Tadasana alignment, inhale, lengthening the spine, and anchor your right hand to your left knee and your left hand to the left side of chair. Variation: If you have lower-back pain, insert a block lengthwise between your thighs.
2. As you exhale, begin the twist from the lower spine, keeping the upper back erect; and, if you feel no pinch or strain, allow the neck to follow.
3. Hold for three for five breaths, lengthening on the inhalations and perhaps deepening the stretch on the exhalations by holding the knee firmly and twisting from the middle and upper back.
4. Inhale and, as you exhale, untwist the spine to return to center.
5. Do the sequence on the left side.
6. Repeat one or two times.

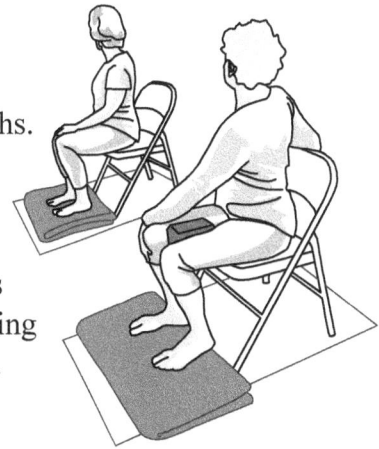

Side-Body Opening

1. Seated in a chair, in Tadasana alignment, anchor your left hand to the side of the chair.
2. Inhaling, sweep your right arm to the side, palm facing up.
3. Exhaling, gently arc the right side-body and arm to the left, rotating the pinky finger toward the floor, without collapsing forward or lifting the right hip.
4. Hold for three to five breaths, perhaps deepening the stretch by lengthening through the arc on the exhalations. If your shoulders are tight, bend the right elbow so that the right hand rests between the shoulder blades.
5. Inhale and, as you exhale, bring your torso upright, sweeping your right arm back to your side, palm facing down.
6. Do the sequence on the other side.
7. Repeat one or two times.

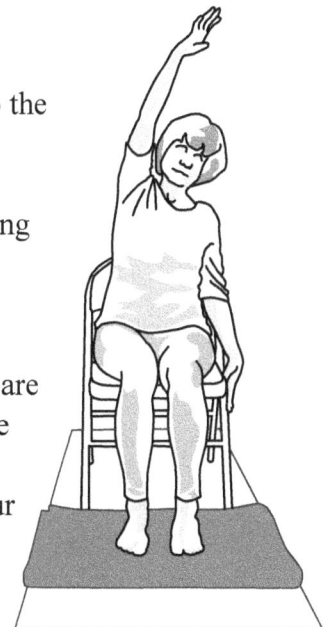

Vakrasana (Twist) Standing

1. Align the long edge of your mat against a wall, and place your chair on the mat, one side of the chair against the wall.
2. Stand in Tadasana alignment, about six inches from the front of the chair, sideways to the wall, facing the seat of the chair.
3. Shifting your weight to the outside leg for stability, place the inside foot fully on the seat of the chair. You may need to adjust the outside foot's distance from the chair so that the inside knee is bent at a 90-degree angle.
4. Place both hands on the wall. On the next inhale, lengthen the body.
5. As you exhale, gently twist toward the wall, pressing into your hands and the foot on the chair for support.
6. Hold for three to five breaths, lengthening on the inhalations, and perhaps deepening the twist on the exhalations.
7. Inhale and, as you exhale, untwist the spine and place the inside foot on the floor, coming back to Tadasana alignment.
8. Turn the chair so that its other side is against the wall, and do the sequence for the other side of your body.
9. Repeat one or two times.

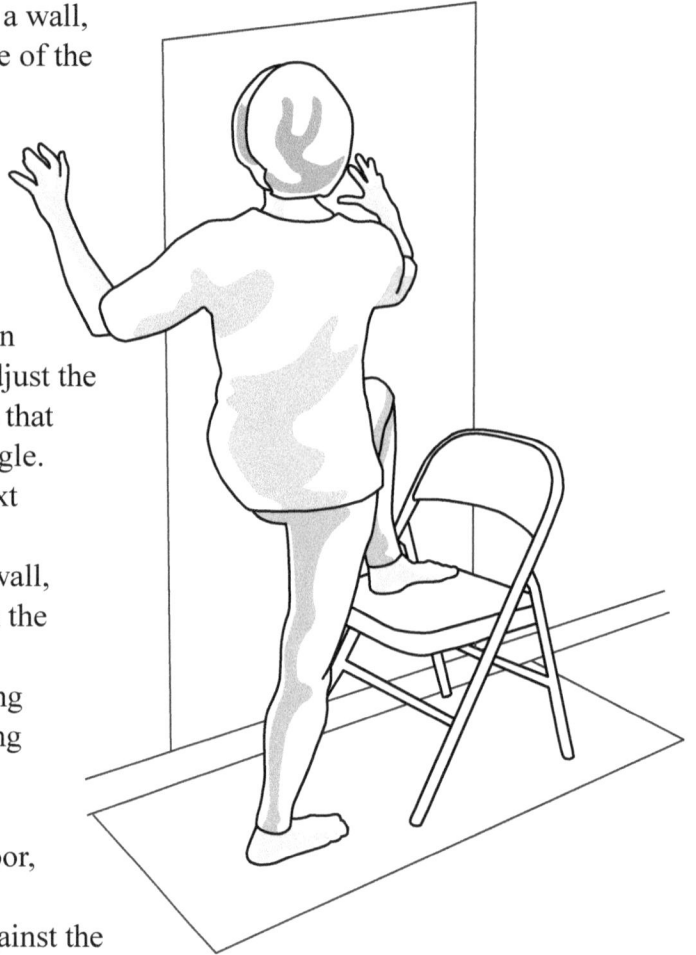

Vakrasana (Twist) Side-Saddle

1. Seated side-saddle on your chair, both feet on the floor, in Tadasana alignment, inhale to lengthen the spine. Variation: If you have lower-back pain, insert a block lengthwise between your thighs.
2. As you exhale, gently twist away from your legs, toward the back of the chair, bringing your hands to Anjali Mudra (p. 11). To twist further, grasp the back of the chair with both hands.
3. Hold for three to five breaths, lengthening on the inhalations and perhaps twisting further on the exhalations.
4. Inhale and, as you exhale, untwist the spine and return to center.
5. Do the sequence on the other side of the chair. Repeat one or two times.

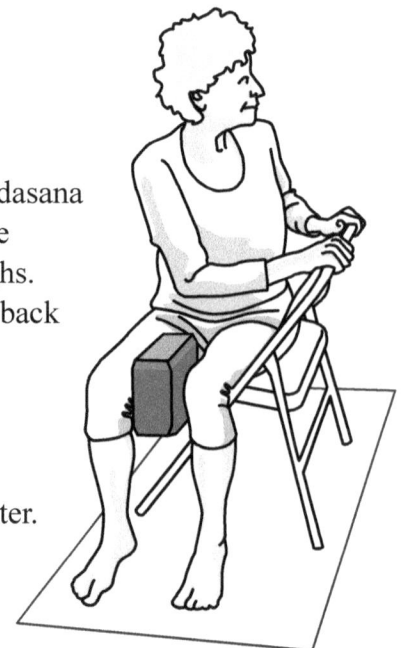

Grateful Virabhadrasana II (Warrior II)

1. While holding Warrior II (pp. 53–54), bring your hands to Anjali Mudra (p. 11).
2. Turn your head to align the chin with the hands. You may bow your head in an expression of respect and gratitude.
3. Hold for three to five breaths.
4. Do the sequence on the other side.
5. Repeat one or two times.

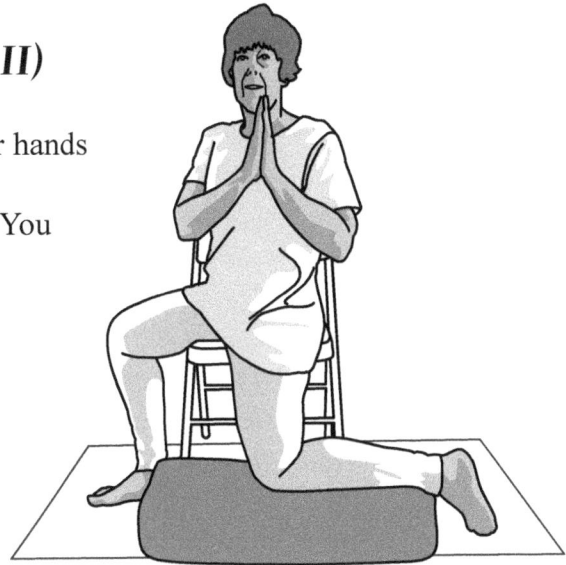

Vakrasana (Twist) Seated with Block

1. Seated in a chair, in Tadasana alignment, place a block just inside the left foot. The lower the block, the deeper the twist, so you may want to position the block at its tallest level or stack two, to start. (Eventually, for an even deeper stretch, place the block just outside the foot.)
2. On the next inhale, lengthen the spine, engaging your core.
3. As you exhale, lower your right hand to the block, looking to the floor, neck in line with the spine, not collapsed. If you feel no pinch or strain in your neck, you may look to the left, right ear parallel to the floor.

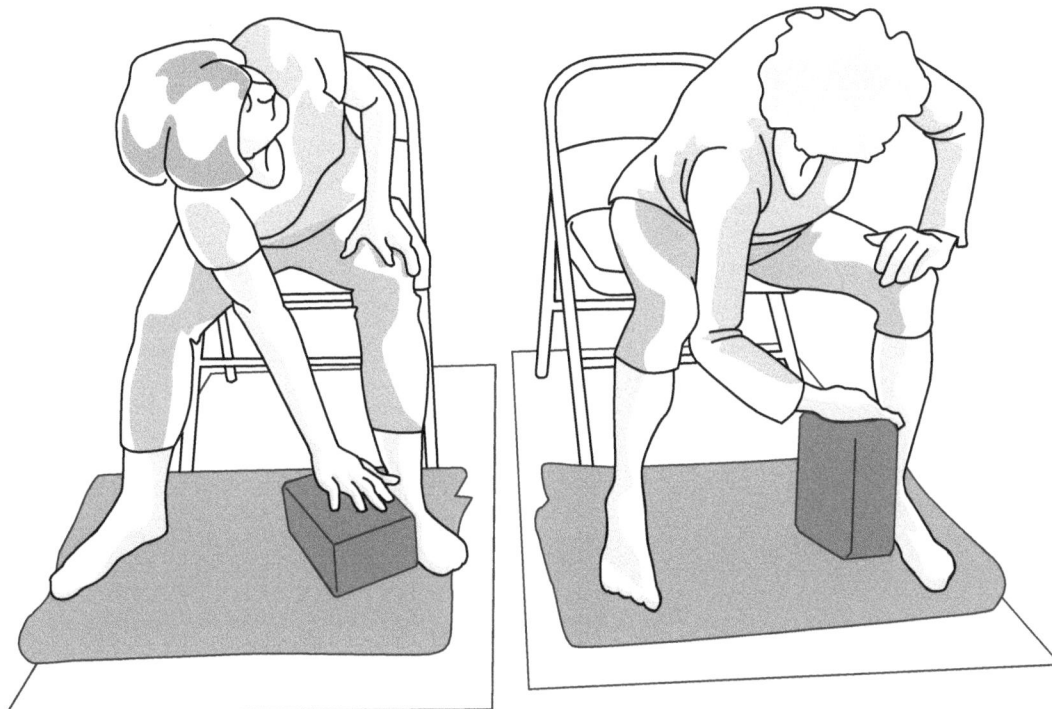

4. Hold for three to five breaths, lengthening on the inhalations and perhaps twisting further on the exhalations.
5. On the next inhale, engaging the core, turn your head to look to the floor and, as you exhale, untwist the spine and bring your torso upright to return to center.
6. Do the sequence on the other side.
7. Repeat one or two times.

Hip Openers

Because tightness or tension in the hips is a common challenge for yoga practitioners, hip openers are among the most frequently requested poses in yoga classes. One contributing factor is the complexity of the musculature around the hips—over twenty muscles, including adductors (inner thigh muscles), responsible for bringing the thighs together; abductors (outer thigh muscles), responsible for bringing the thighs apart; hip flexors, including the psoas (muscles connecting the femurs to the pelvis and lumbar spine), responsible for bringing the knees to the chest and bending at the waist; and the medial and lateral rotators (muscles connecting the femurs to the pelvis and sacrum), responsible, respecively, for internal and external rotation. Another contributor is the notion that the hips store negative feelings and unresolved emotions, especially those related to control.

Benefits:
- Increase mobility and flexibility
- Stretch and strengthen the muscles of the hip
- Improve range of motion and circulation, which decreases the load on the spine, thereby lessening overuse and the resultant back pain
- Release physical, emotional, and energetic tension
- Create space for decision-making: new ideas, new pathways, even new beginnings
- Promote freedom in the body and in our unique creative, physical, and spiritual expression

Abductors and Adductors

1. Seated in a chair, in Tadasana alignment, place the palm of one hand on top of the same-side knee.
2. Lift that leg up, a few inches off the floor, and move it to the inside, then to the outside, keeping the other foot on the floor and gently pressing your palm on your knee for resistance.
3. Do the back-and-forth movement for three to five breaths.
4. Do the sequence on the other side.
5. Repeat one or two times.

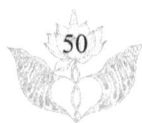

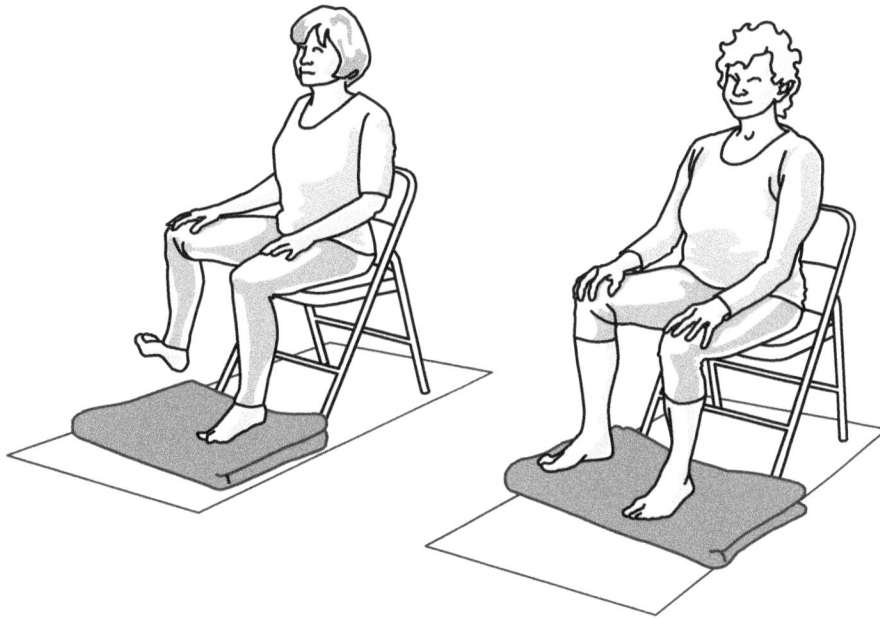

Baddha Konasana (Butterfly)

1. Seated in a chair, in Tadasana alignment, place a block under each sole, at the height most comfortable for your body.
2. Bring your soles together, allowing the knees to splay out.
3. Stay here and enjoy the stretch or, to deepen the stretch, engage your core and slowly bend forward, keeping your back as straight as possible.
4. Hold for three to five breaths.
5. With your back straight and your core engaged, slowly bring your torso upright.
6. Repeat one or two times.

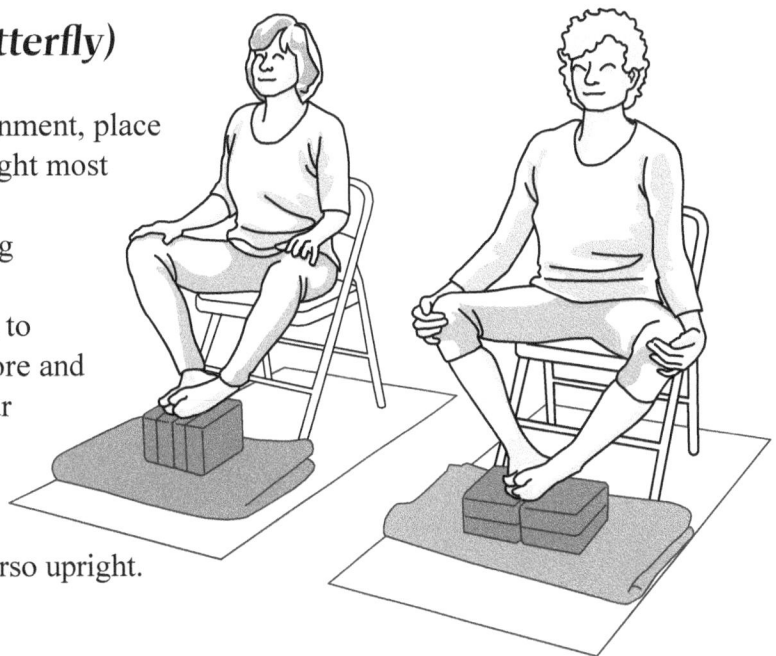

Straight-Leg Abductor and Adductor

1. Seated in a chair, in Tadasana alignment, wrap a yoga strap under the sole of one foot. If your back needs support, insert a rolled mat or block between the chair and your back.
2. Straighten that leg as much as is comfortable, keeping a slight bend in the knee.
3. Once you have found that stretch, slowly move your leg out to the side, then back to center, back and forth for three to five breaths.
4. Do the sequence with the other leg.
5. Repeat one or two times.

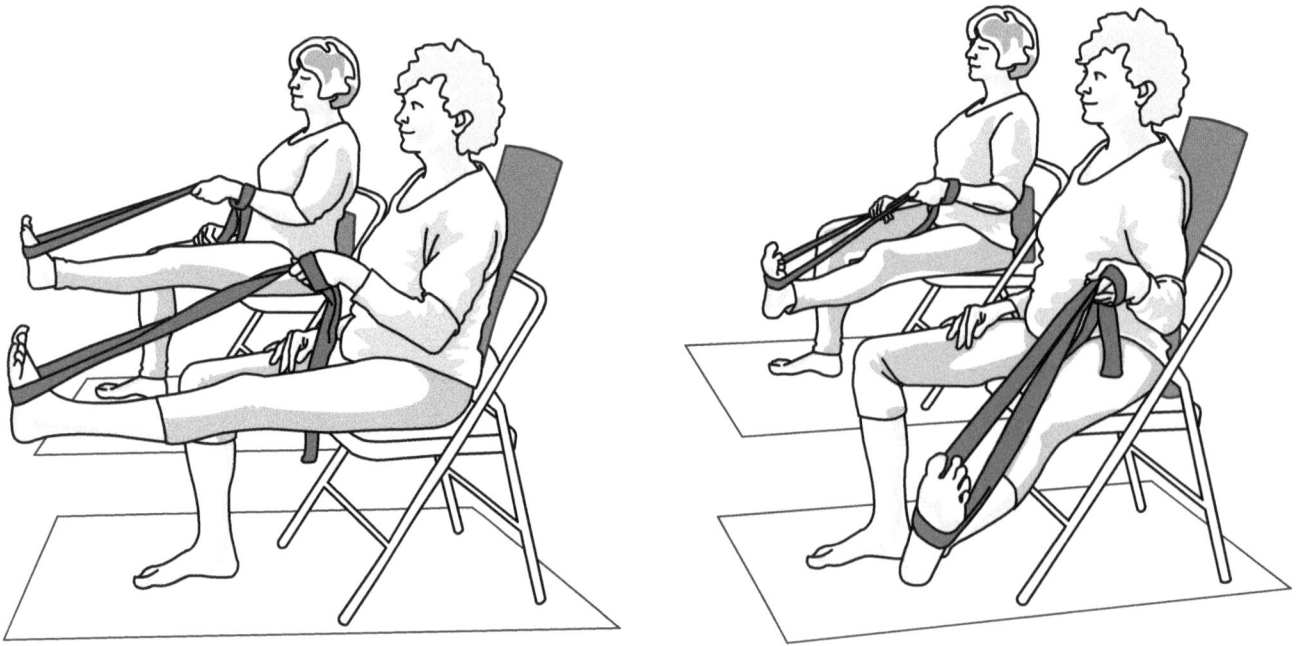

Kapotasana (Pigeon)

1. Seated in a chair, in Tadasana alignment, cross your ankle over the other knee, keeping the hips square and the other foot planted. If crossing the ankle over the knee is challenging, cross your foot over the other ankle or rest it on a block placed just outside the planted foot. Either way, flex the ankle so that your toes point toward the knee, to protect the knee. If your back needs support, insert a rolled mat or block between the chair and your back.
2. Stay here and enjoy the stretch or, to deepen the stretch, engage your core and slowly bend forward, keeping your back as straight as possible.
3. Hold for three to five breaths.
4. With your back straight and your core engaged, slowly bring your torso upright.
5. Do the sequence with the other leg. Repeat one or two times.

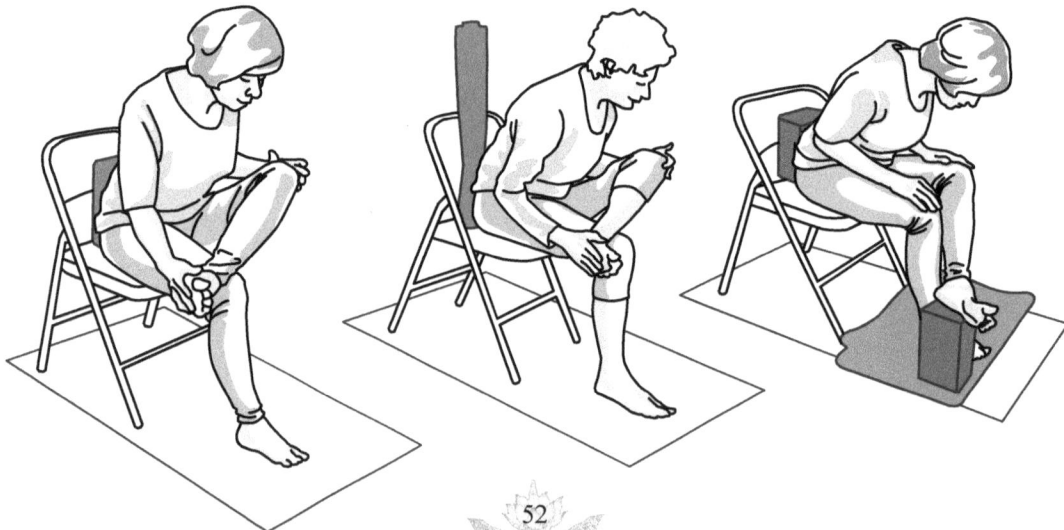

Knee Circles

1. Seated in a chair, in Tadasana alignment, lift the right knee so that your foot is six inches from the floor.
2. Circle your knee to the inside for three to five breaths, then to the outside for three to five breaths.
3. Shake the right leg to release tension, and return that foot to the floor.
4. Do the sequence with the left knee.
5. Repeat one or two times.

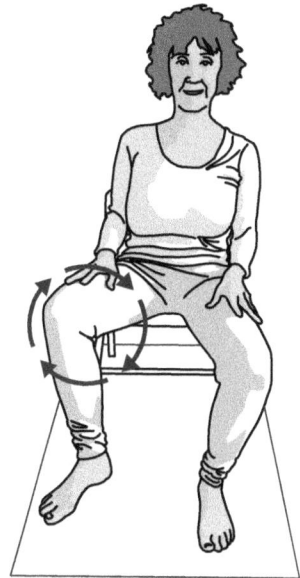

Virabhadrasana I (Warrior I)

1. Place a bolster, pillow, or rolled blanket in front of your yoga chair, with the long side up against the chair's front legs.
2. Sit sideways in the chair, in Tadasana alignment, feet parallel and hip-width apart on the floor.
3. Keeping the inside foot planted, place your outside knee on the bolster to come into a lunge. Both legs should be bent at a 90-degree angle, inside knee directly over inside ankle, outside hip directly over outside knee.
4. Keeping your alignment, bring your hands to Anjali Mudra (p. 11), and gaze toward where the wall and ceiling meet. Keep the neck long and the shoulders back and down, away from the ears. If it is comfortable for your shoulders, raise your arms to a goalpost position or fully overhead.
5. Hold this posture, moving in and out of various arm positions, for three to five breaths.
6. Do the sequence on the opposite side.
7. Repeat one or two times.

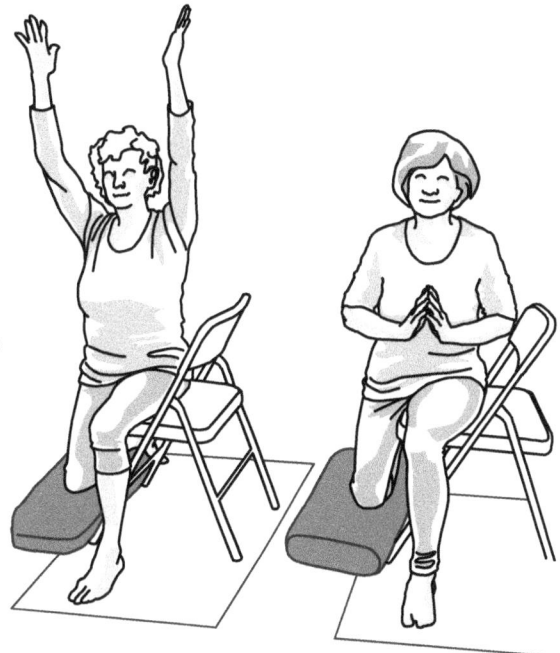

Virabhadrasana II (Warrior II)

1. While holding Warrior I (above), forward-extend the same-side arm as the front leg, palm down; and back-extend the other arm, palm down.

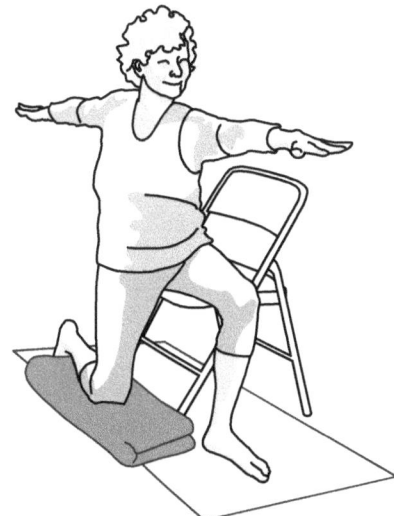

2. Turn your upper body away from the back of the chair, and gaze over your front hand, lengthening your body from front fingertips to back fingertips.
3. Hold for three to five breaths.
4. Do the sequence on the other side.
5. Repeat one or two times.

Viparita Virabhadrasana (Reverse Warrior)

1. While holding Warrior I (p. 53), bring the hand of the bolstered knee to the same-side thigh, front, side, or back.
2. Sliding your hand to the lower thigh, gently arch your back, lifting your heart, keeping the neck aligned with the spine, and gaze toward where the wall and ceiling meet.
3. Reach your other arm to the ceiling, palm facing inward, or place that hand on your heart. If the back, neck, or shoulders experience any strain, ease up on the posture.
4. Hold for three to five breaths.
5. Do the sequence on the other side.
6. Repeat one or two times.

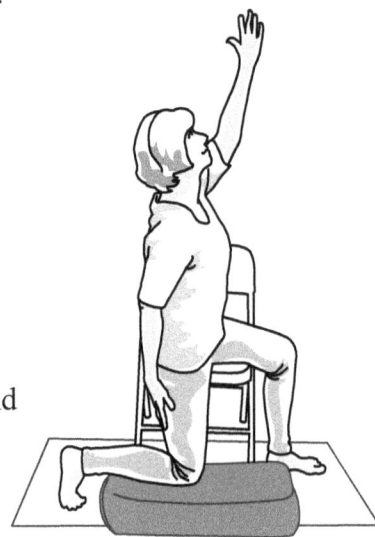

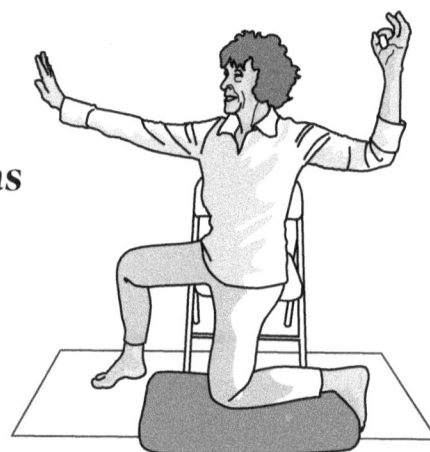

Virabhadrasana II (Warrior II) with Mudras

1. While holding Warrior II (pp. 53–54), bring your front hand into Abhaya Mudra (p. 12).
2. Bend your back arm at the elbow, and bring that hand into Gyan Mudra (p. 11).
3. Lift the heel of the front foot.
4. Hold for three to five breaths.
5. Do the sequence on the other side.
6. Repeat one or two times.

Utthita Parsvakonasana (Extended Warrior)

1. While holding Warrior II (pp. 53–54), bring your front elbow to your front knee.
2. Inhaling, extend your back arm up toward the ceiling, palm rotated toward the body.
3. Exhaling, bring the extended arm toward the ear. Feel the side-body open from the pinky toe to the pinky finger.
4. Hold for three to five breaths.
5. Inhaling, rotate the extended palm toward the ceiling and, exhaling, return both arms to Warrior II.

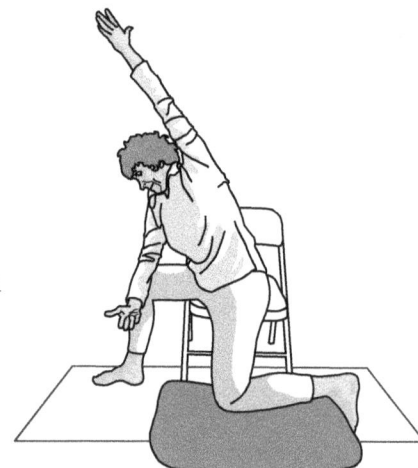

6. Do the sequence on the other side.
7. Repeat one or two times.

Virabhadrasana (Warrior) Flow

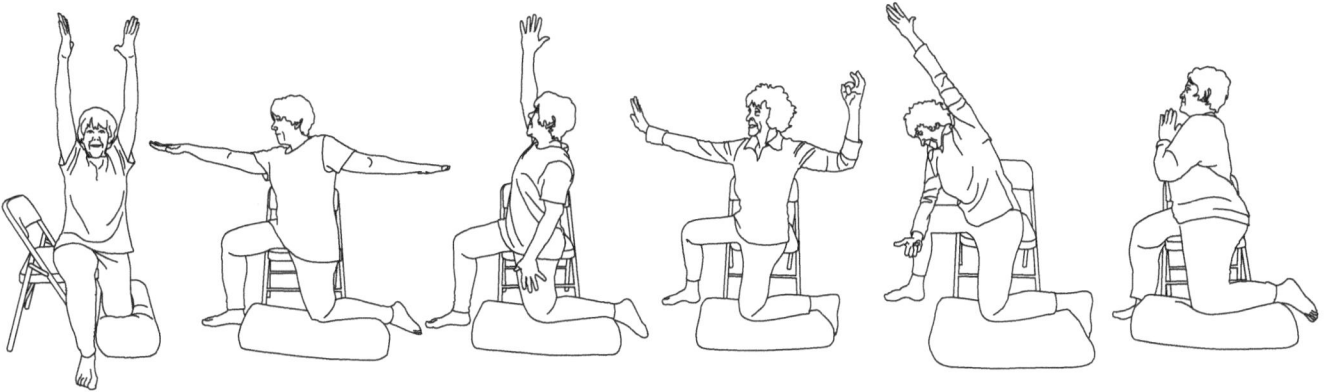

1. While holding Warrior I (p. 53), with your hands in Anjali Mudra (p. 11) or your arms in a goalpost position or fully overhead, take three to five breaths.
2. Transition to Warrior II (pp. 53–54). Hold for three to five breaths.
3. Transition to Reverse Warrior (p. 54). Hold for three to five breaths.
4. Transition to Warrior II with Mudras (p. 54). Hold for three to five breaths.
5. Transition to Extended Warrior (pp. 54–55). Hold for three to five breaths.
6. Return to Warrior I, with your hands in Anjali Mudra, and bow your head.
7. Do the sequence on the other side.

Supta Padangusthasana (Big-Toe Stretch)

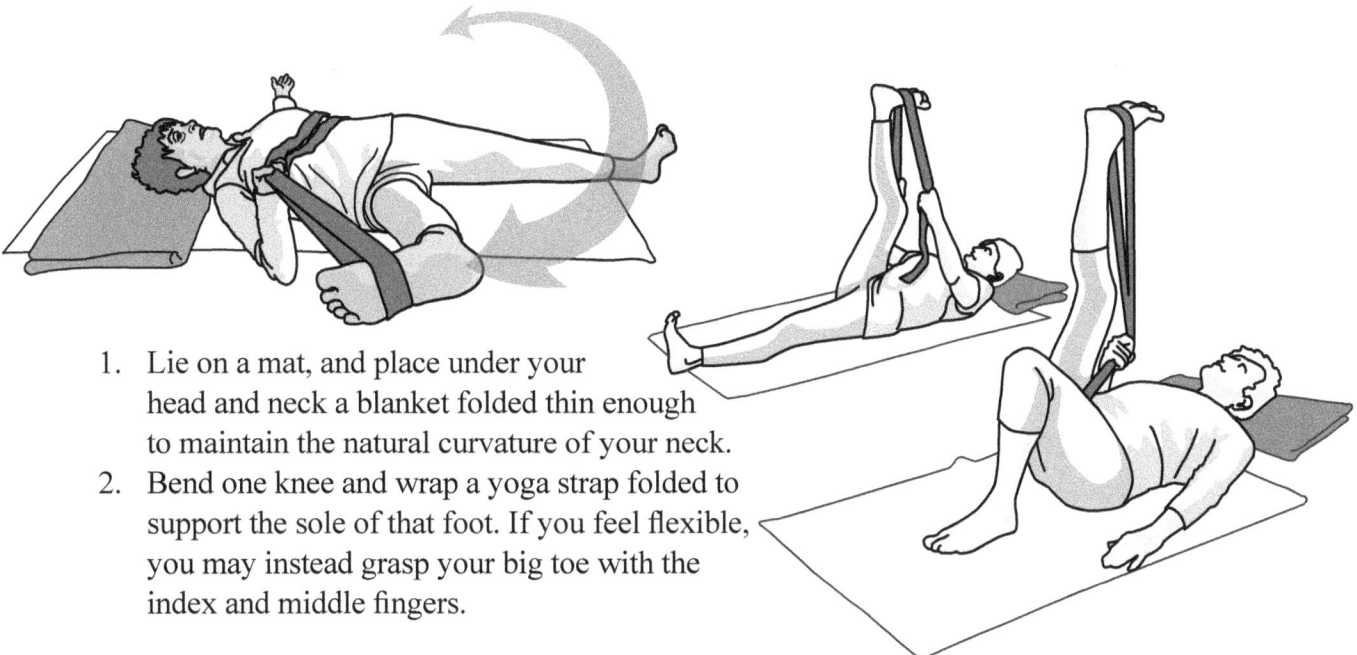

1. Lie on a mat, and place under your head and neck a blanket folded thin enough to maintain the natural curvature of your neck.
2. Bend one knee and wrap a yoga strap folded to support the sole of that foot. If you feel flexible, you may instead grasp your big toe with the index and middle fingers.

3. Holding an end of the strap in each hand, extend that leg toward the ceiling slowly, so as not to strain the hamstring muscle. Press into the heel, toes toward your body, keeping a slight bend in the knee.
4. Grab both ends of the strap in the same-side hand of the extended leg, and allow the leg to fall out to the outside, keeping the other hip anchored. You may place a bolster under the extended foot.
5. Slightly bend the knee of the extended leg, and bring the leg to center.
6. Grab both ends of the strap in the other hand. Bring the extended leg across your body into a gentle spinal twist.
7. Hold for three to five breaths.
8. Do the sequence with the other leg.
9. Repeat one or two times.

Balance

Movement is inherent in balance. The body's constant give-and-take to retain posture and stability involves our front and back bodies, as well as the many small muscles throughout our body. Balance asks us to be in the now, mindful of where we are stepping without having to look at the ground. Coming to balance in asanas, we discover that we are not rigid and unmoving but always in flux, bending and wobbling, stabilizing our body through movement.

Benefits:
- Fosters physical equilibrium and steadiness
- Improves posture and coordination
- Strengthens the ankles, legs, and glutes
- Increases mental focus and mindfulness
- Supports emotional steadiness

Foot Massage

1. Seated in a chair, in Tadasana alignment, cross your foot over the opposite knee.
2. Use your opposite hand to gently massage the entire foot, from toes to heel.
3. Interlace the fingers with the toes as if you are holding hands with your foot—pinky finger under the base of the little toe, ring finger slid under the base of the next toe, and so on, until your fingers and toes are firmly connected, thumb on top of the big toe.
4. Gently spread your fingers as wide apart as you can.
5. Hold for three to five breaths.
6. Do the sequence with the other foot.
7. Repeat one or two times. (Five minutes of this asana alone will help stimulate the connective tissue via marma points.)

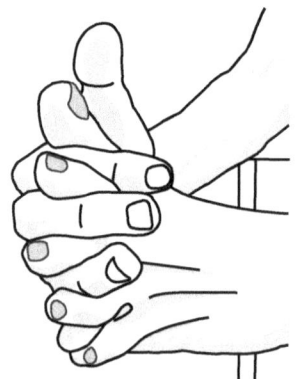

On Your Toes

1. Standing directly behind a chair, in Tadasana alignment, hold the back of the chair with both hands.
2. Inhaling, rise on the tiptoes.
3. Exhaling, lower your feet to the floor and rock back on the heels, toes lifted.
4. Repeat for three to five breaths, in a continuous flow.
5. Return to standing and shake out each foot.
6. Repeat one or two times.

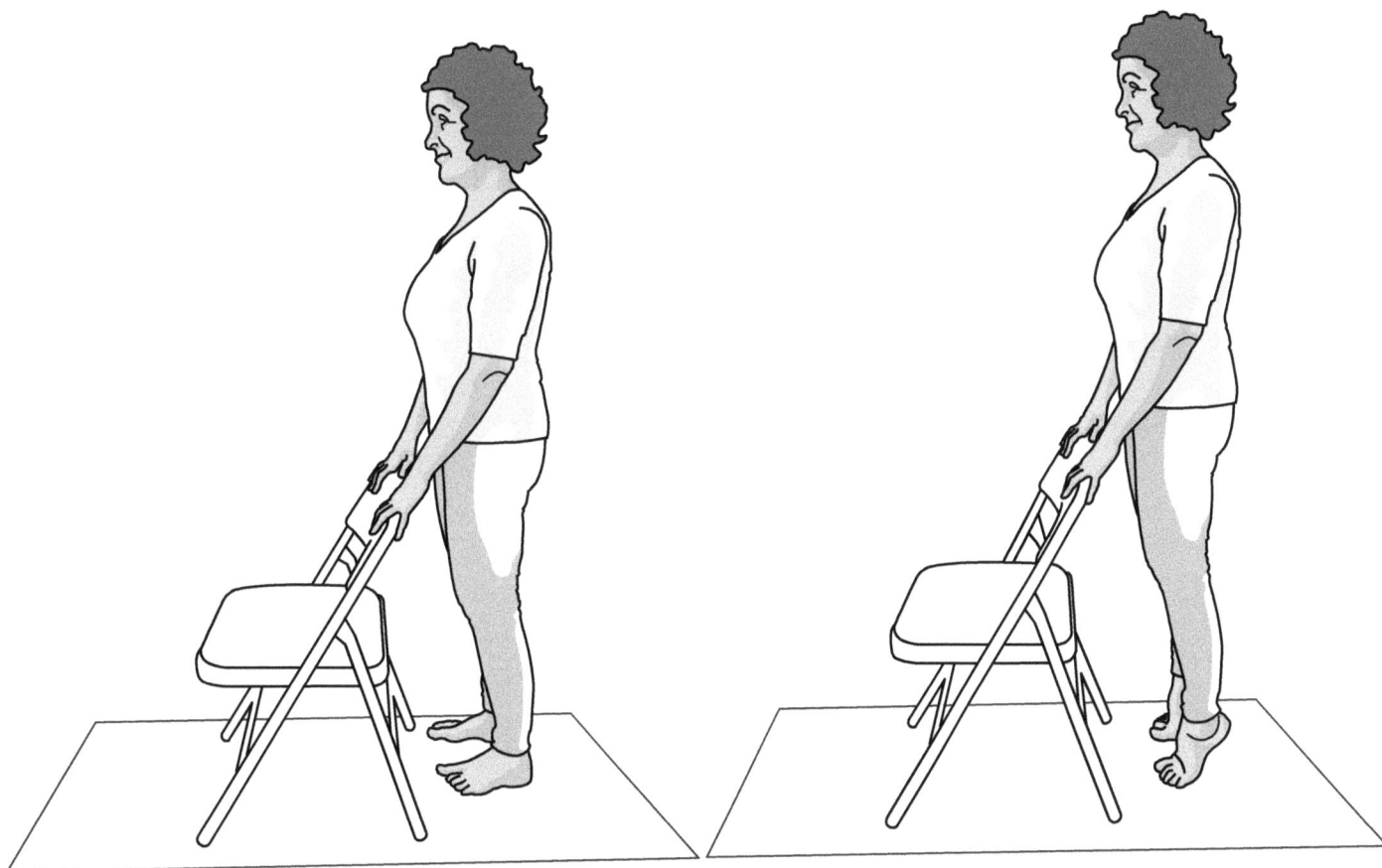

Wall Stretch

1. Align the short edge of your mat against a wall.
2. Stand facing the wall, eight to twelve inches from it, in Tadasana alignment.
3. Stretch your arms up, shoulder-width apart, and place your fingertips on the wall so that your hands look like Daddy Long Legs.
4. Inhaling, rise on the tiptoes, lengthening your arms and torso farther up the wall, core engaged.

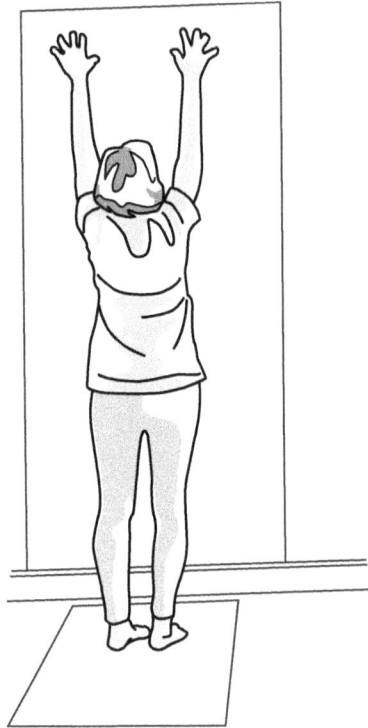

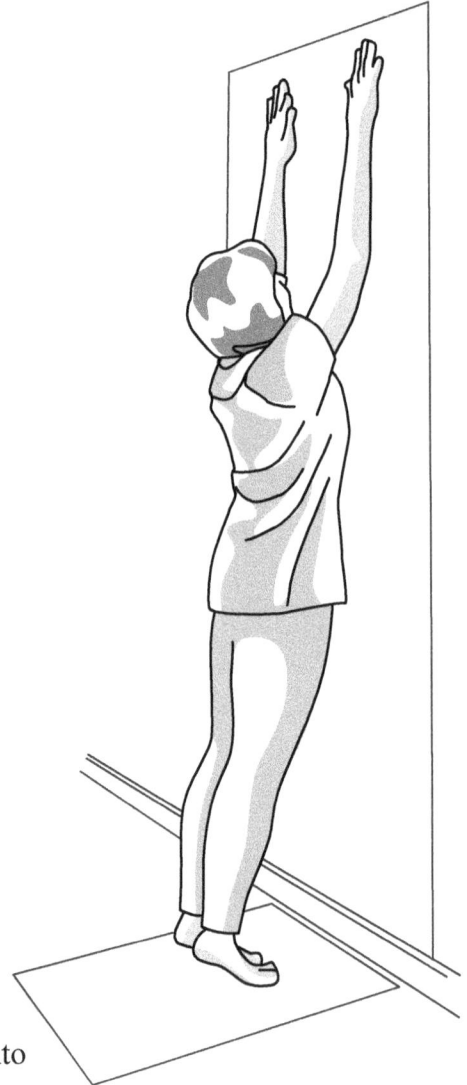

5. Exhaling into the back-body, slowly lower your feet to the floor, dropping your shoulders down and together, maintaining the positioning of your fingertips as much as possible.

6. Engaging your core, gently push the fingertips into the wall such that your body weight redistributes over the heels without lifting the toes.

7. Hold for three to five breaths, feeling the stretch.

8. Relax your arms at the sides, realigning your body into an upright position, perhaps closing your eyes.

9. Repeat one or two times.

Vriksasana (Tree)

1. Align the long edge of your mat against a wall, and place a chair sideways against the wall.

2. Stand behind the chair at a distance that allows you to hold the back of the chair while maintaining Tadasana alignment.

3. Distribute your weight evenly across your feet, and draw energy up from the ground.

4. Bring the outside foot to the inside ankle such that the outside knee splays to the side. You may keep your toes on the floor or raise them either to the ankle, just below the knee, just above the knee, or even to the inner thigh—wherever you feel steady. Do not place the foot directly on the knee.

5. If you feel balanced, let go of the chair and bring your hands to prayer pose at heart

center or above the head. If you do not feel balanced, bring only the outside arm up.

6. Hold for three to five breaths at first, eventually working up to one minute.
7. Do the sequence on the other side.
8. Repeat one or two times.
9. Variation for #1–2: Align the short edge of your mat against a wall, and stand in Tadasana alignment such that your back lightly rests against the wall.

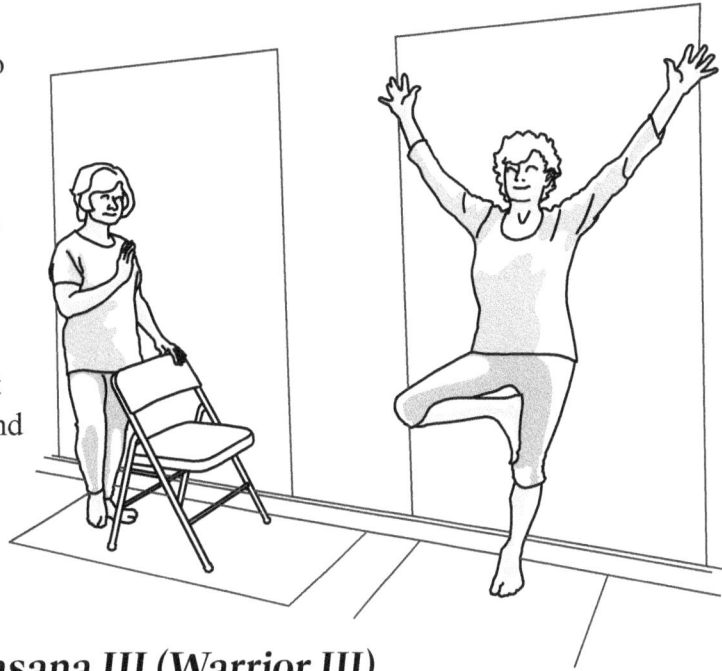

Virabhadrasana III (Warrior III)

1. Stand behind a chair, in Tadasana alignment. Bring both hands over the back of the chair to rest on the seat, shoulder-width apart.
2. Extend your left leg back and up, no higher than hip level, toes pointing to the floor, upper body bending from the hip, core engaged, until it forms a straight line with that leg. Keep the standing leg as straight as you can without locking the knee.
3. If you feel balanced, extend your right arm forward, aligned with the ear.
4. Hold for three to five breaths, lengthening from the left heel to the right fingertips, keeping the core engaged.
5. Gently lower your hand to the chair and your foot to the floor.
6. Do the sequence on the other side.
7. Repeat one or two times.

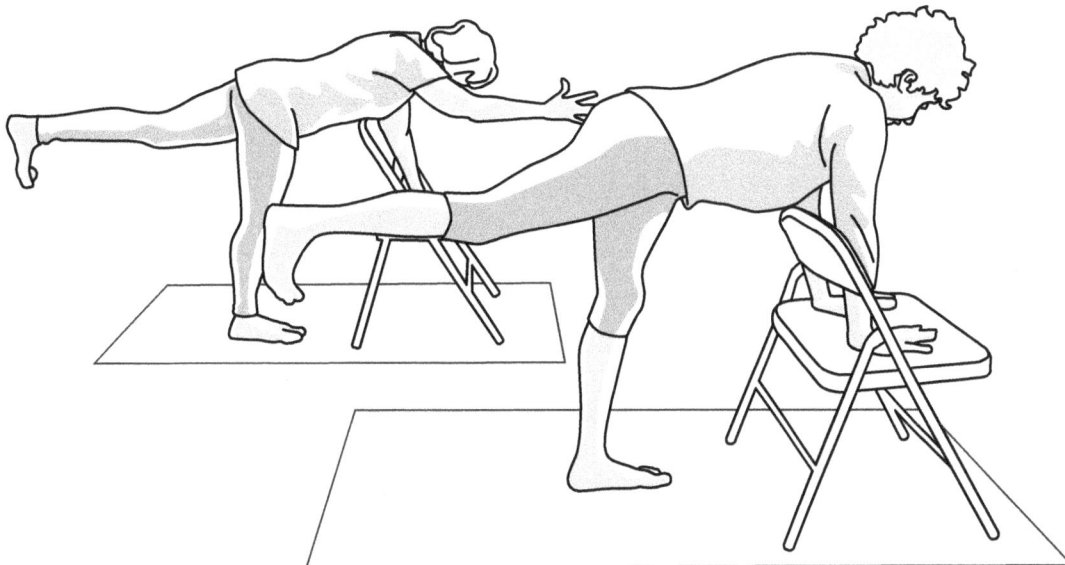

Ardha Chandrasana (Half Moon)

1. Align the short edge of your mat against a wall, and place the back of a chair against the wall, with a block on the seat to have handy.
2. Stand sideways about six inches from the chair, in Tadasana alignment.
3. Place your inside foot entirely on the seat, knee at a 90-degree angle, toes pointing toward the wall.
4. Inhaling, place your inside hand on the wall or, if you need the surface closer, on the block. Lengthen through the spine and neck.
5. Exhaling, raise your outside arm parallel to the floor, palm down. If you feel balanced and flexible, raise your arm straight overhead, palm facing the wall; or, for a deeper stretch, arc your arm over your head, pinky finger rotated toward the body.
6. Hold for three to five breaths, lengthening from the outside foot to the fingertips.
7. Palm down, return the outside arm to your side. Remove the block under the inside palm, and bring the inside leg to the floor.
8. Do the sequence on the other side.
9. Repeat one or two times.

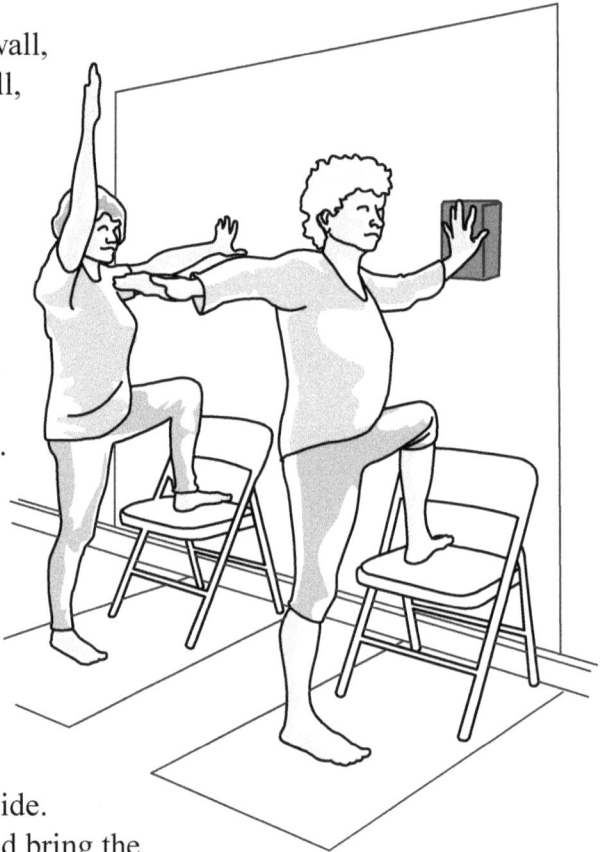

Garudasana (Eagle)

1. Align the short edge of your mat against a wall, and stand in Tadasana alignment such that your back lightly rests against the wall. Place a block at the outer edge of your left foot, if needed in #5.
2. Inhaling, lengthen the spine and extend your arms to the sides at shoulder level.
3. Exhaling, cross your right arm under the left arm, aligning the elbows, and bend the elbows until your hands align, fingers pointing toward the ceiling.
4. Place your right fingers into your left palm, pressing your two hands together. If your hands can't quite touch like that yet, press the backs of the hands together or simply place the left palm on the right shoulder and the right palm on the left shoulder.
5. Cross your right ankle over the left ankle, and rest your right foot or toes on the mat or block. If you feel balanced and flexible, wrap your right foot behind the left calf.
6. Gently lift your elbows, reaching the fingertips toward the ceiling if they are not on the shoulders.

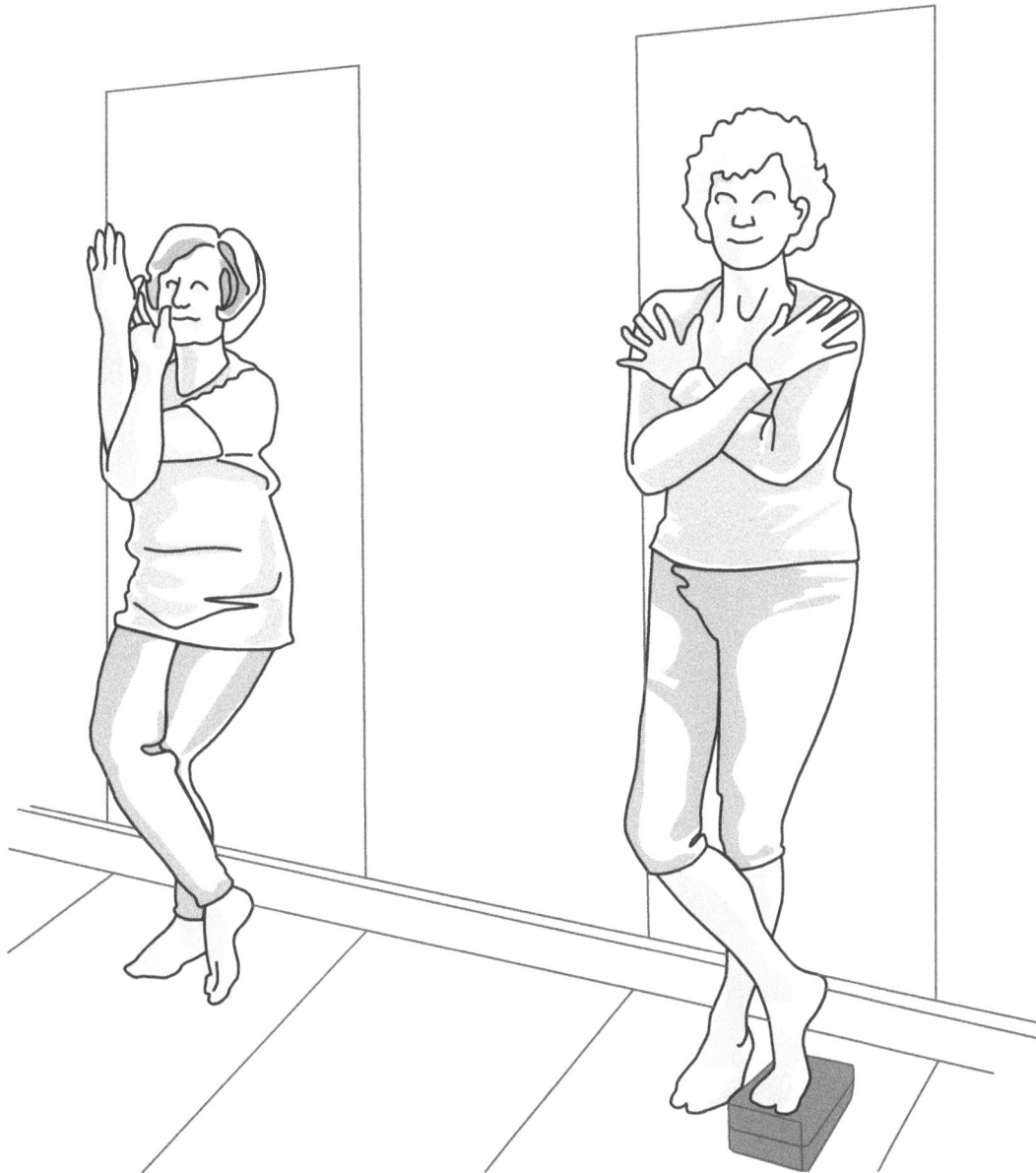

7. Hold for three to five breaths, focusing on the inhalations and exhalations, and keeping your gaze fixed and soft.
8. Unwind your arms and legs, and gently shake them out.
9. Do the sequence on the other side, left arm under right arm, left ankle over right ankle, moving the block, if needed, to the outer edge of your right foot.
10. Repeat one or two times.
11. Variation: If, after #6, you feel balanced, slowly move your head forward, six to twelve inches from the wall; your shoulders and back will follow. Keep your buttocks anchored to the wall. Bend your knees to deepen the pose.

Natarajasana (Dancer)

1. Place the front of a chair against the wall, and stand directly behind the chair, facing the wall, in Tadasana alignment.
2. Hold the back of the chair with your right hand; or, if you need more support, place your right hand on the wall.
3. Slide your left hand down your left leg, and, bending that knee, gently grasp the ankle or wrap a yoga strap around the ankle.
4. If your knee feels no pain or strain, gently bring the heel back toward your buttocks until the knee is pointed toward the floor.
5. Hold for three to five breaths.

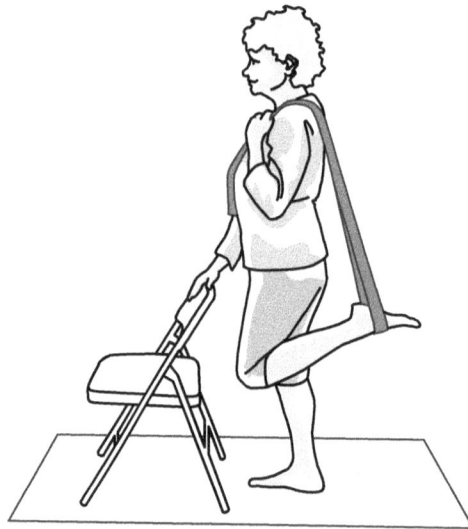

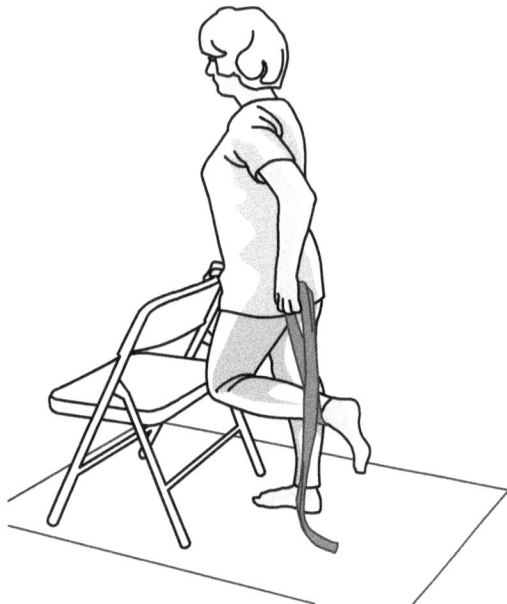

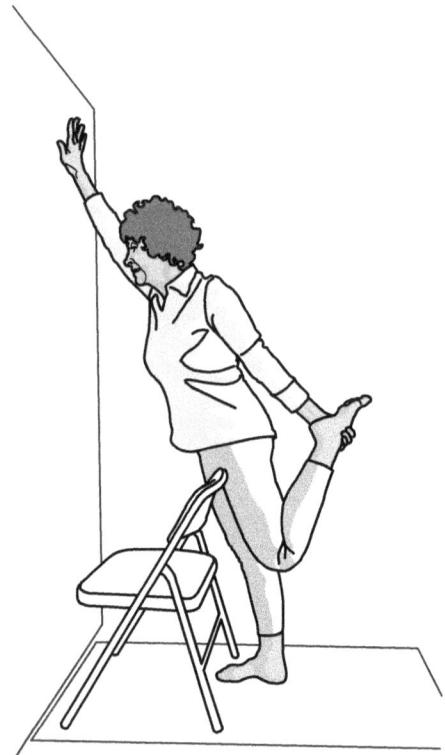

6. Gently release your ankle.
7. Do the sequence on the other side.
8. Repeat one or two times.
9. Variation: If, after #4, you feel balanced, lift your stabilizing hand from the chair or away from the wall and, if possible, press your ankle away from the buttocks.

These asanas move and groove the body to keep our muscles, ligaments, and joints lubricated, flexible, and strong. Our physical vitality grounds and extends our mental and emotional well-being, too.

Now let's relax, restore, and cool down the body with restorative asanas.

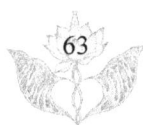

Yoga transforms the here and now,
wherever and whenever you are.
~Linda Anastasia Ransom

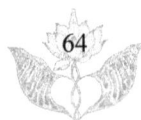

CHAPTER IV

Cooling Down: Restorative Asanas

Restorative yoga, sometimes referred to as active relaxation, can be a part of your daily practice or an occasional separate practice. The latter typically involves three or four asanas, held for fifteen to twenty minutes each, supported by props to allow the body to fully let go, to restore itself to all-over balance and harmony. As part of a total-body practice, one restorative asana may be added, held for five to ten minutes.

Restorative asanas, based on the teachings of B.K.S. Iyengar, include light twists, seated forward folds, inversions, and gentle backbends. These poses passively stretch your muscles, lower your heart rate and blood pressure, calm your nervous system, and move your body into a peaceful state of deep relaxation.

Stillness and restfulness, however, may arouse unease or anxiety for some of us, some of the time—which does not mean you shouldn't do restorative yoga! These are exactly the times when you can most benefit from its soothing therapeutic function, practicing for five to ten minutes and building up from there. Restorative yoga is especially helpful before, during, and after major life events and when you're unable to maintain your regular yoga practice due to illness, injury, or pregnancy.

Precaution: If you are pregnant or have high blood pressure or glaucoma, consult your doctor before adding inversions to your yoga practice—poses in which the heart is higher from the ground than the head. This chapter includes two inversions: Babbling Mountain Brook (pp. 71–72) and Setu Bandha Sarvangasana (p. 73). The modified Viparita Karani poses (pp. 69–70 and p. 77) and Supta Baddha Konasana variations (pp. 66–68 and pp. 70–71) in this chapter and in Chapter V are not inversions because these asanas are demonstrated with the heart and head positioned at the same level. However, if you are unsure, consult your doctor before practicing these poses.

May you be inspired to include at least one restorative asana in your daily practice, or to devote one entire practice each week or each month to restorative yoga.

Benefits:
- Stimulate and soothe the organs
- Reduce levels of cortisol, the stress hormone
- Relieve the effects of chronic stress
- Mitigate the sympathetic nervous system, the fight-or-flight response, and activate the parasympathetic nervous system, the rest-and-digest state
- Boost one's mood and ease fatigue
- Improve the quality of sleep
- Redistribute blood and lymph fluid from the lower extremities to the upper body
- Relieve chronic health conditions, such as headaches, back pain, and genetic diseases
- Balance the body's masculine energy (*prana*), which moves upward from the diaphragm, and the feminine energy (*apana*), which moves downward from the diaphragm

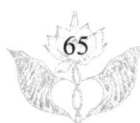

Before coming into a restorative pose, be sure to have all your props, including an extra blanket to cover yourself once you're in the pose. To further stay warm, you might also wear socks and a sweater. To further relax, you might cover your eyes with the eyebag. Choose a pranayama—Ujjayi (p. 8) and Dirga (p. 9) are suggested—and a mudra (pp. 11–12) that matches the intention you may wish to focus the breath on.

Supta Baddha Konasana (Bound Angle) in Chair

1. Gather your props: a chair, a mat, two blocks, two bolsters, and two blankets.
2. Align the short edge of your mat against a wall, and place the chair on the mat, with its back against the wall.
3. Place the two blocks hip-width apart in front of your chair, vertically at their lowest height (higher if it feels better for your body); and place a bolster horizontally on top of the blocks. For additional support, place a bolster vertically between the chair and your back, and place a blanket between the bolster and your head.

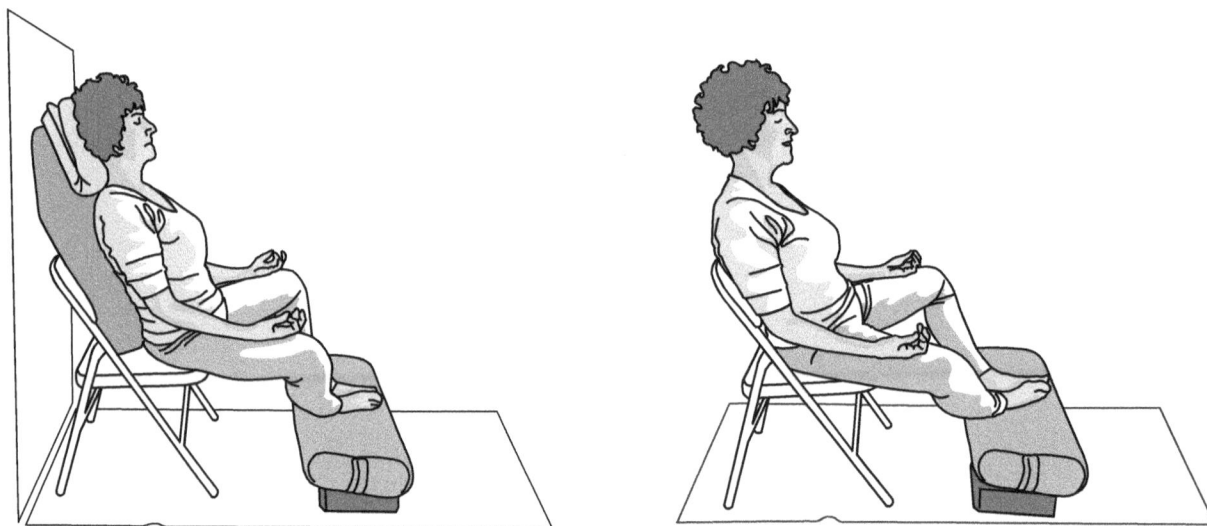

4. Bring your soles together, allowing the knees to splay out.
5. Place your hands on your thighs, palms up or down, fingers positioned in a mudra if you like.
6. Close your eyes, relax your entire body, and breathe into the pose for fifteen to twenty minutes (or until you are ready to come out of it). Feel your heart, stomach, and pelvis open.

Supta Baddha Konasana (Bound Angle) Reclining with Chair

1. Gather your props: a chair, a mat, two blocks, one bolster, three blankets, and an eyebag (optional).
2. Align the short edge of the mat against a wall, and place the chair on the mat, with its back against the wall for safety.

3. Place a blanket, folded in half, horizontally on the mat, aligned with the chair.
4. Lie on the mat, facing the chair seat, and place your feet on the chair so that your soles touch and your knees splay out in Bound Angle Pose. You may need to shift your buttocks closer to or farther from the chair.
5. Notice where your lower back meets the mat, just above the pelvis: this is where one end of the bolster will go. Roll to your side and come to a seated position.
6. Position the bolster vertically, with the bottom end where your lower back had been, and place the two blocks under the bolster as follows: the first block, horizontally at its medium height, at least halfway up the bolster; the second block, at its highest height, between the first block and the top end of the bolster.
7. Place a blanket on the bolster where your head and neck will rest, folded thin enough to maintain the natural curvature of the neck.

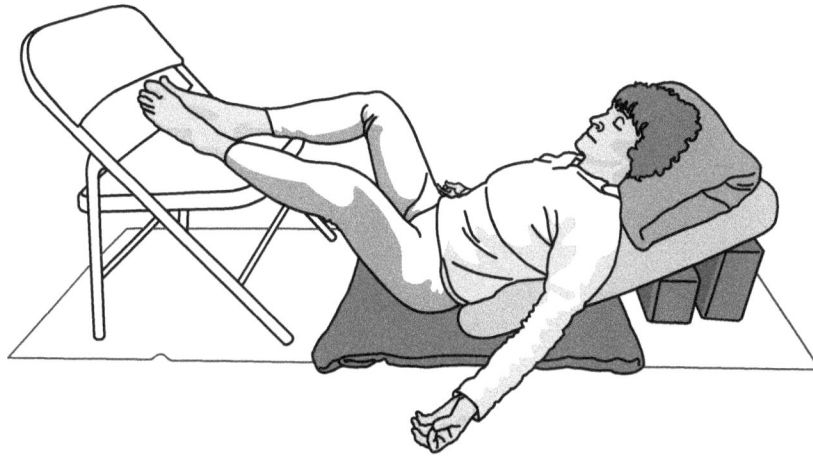

8. Again, lie on the mat, facing the chair seat, and place your feet on the chair so that your soles touch and your knees splay out in Bound Angle Pose. You might place a blanket on the chair for cushion or warmth.
9. Bring your arms out to the side at a 45-degree angle, palms up, or place your hands on your belly, fingers positioned in a mudra if you like. Adjust the blocks for greater stability, if needed.
10. Close your eyes (or cover them with the eyebag), relax your entire body and breathe into the pose for fifteen to twenty minutes (or until you are ready to come out of it). Feel your chest, abdomen, and hips open.

Supta Baddha Konasana (Bound Angle) with Two Chairs

1. Gather your props: two chairs, a mat, two blocks, one bolster, one blanket, and an eyebag (optional). You may need to use two regular chairs (not folding chairs) to better accommodate the range of motion of your hips.
2. Align the short edge of the mat against a wall, and place both chairs on the mat, one with its back against the wall for safety, and the other about six inches from the first chair, seats facing each other.

3. Place the two blocks on the first chair's seat as follows: the first block, horizontally at its lowest height; the second block, vertically on top of the first block, with the larger side facing out.
4. Place the bolster vertically over the blocks so that the bottom end rests on the edge of the second chair's seat; and place the blanket on the bolster where your head and neck will rest, folded thin enough to maintain the natural curvature of the neck.
5. Straddle the second chair's seat, facing its seat-back, feet planted, and lie back slowly so that the props stay in place.
6. Place your hands on your belly, fingers positioned in a mudra if you like.
7. Close your eyes (or cover them with the eyebag), relax your entire body, and breathe into the pose for fifteen to twenty minutes (or until you are ready to come out of it). Feel your heart and front body open in full trust.
8. Precaution: If you have a hip condition, consult your doctor before practicing this pose.

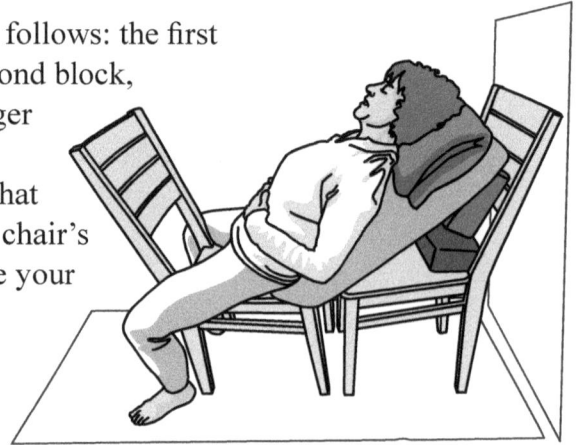

Uttanasana (Forward Fold) Big Hug with Two Chairs

1. Gather your props: two chairs, a mat, one block, and one bolster.
2. Align the short edge of the mat against a wall, and place both chairs on the mat, one with its back against the wall for safety, and the other six to eight inches from the first chair, seats facing each other.
3. Place the block vertically on the second chair's seat so that it leans against the seat-back; and place the bolster vertically, at a 45-degree angle, so that the bottom end rests on the edge of the first chair's seat and the top end rests against the block.
4. Straddle the first chair's seat, facing the second chair, feet planted, and bow forward to wrap your arms around the bolster, resting the forearms on the seat, between the bolster and the block.
5. Turn your head to the right and rest it on the bolster for five minutes; then turn your head to left and rest it on the bolster for five minutes; then rest your forehead on the bolster for five minutes. For each head placement, close your eyes, relax your entire body, and breathe into the pose for the specified time (or until you are ready to come out of it). Feel your back body stretch and open, as if surrendering into a big hug.
6. Variation for #5: Turn your head to the side that feels best for your neck, and remain in this position for the entire fifteen minutes (or until you are ready to come out of it).

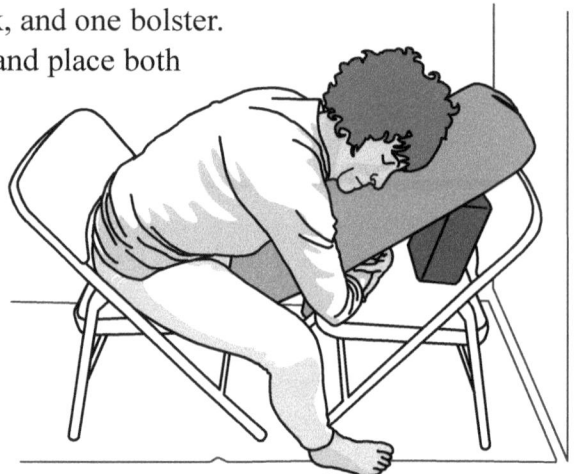

If your neck feels strained or pinched, rest your forehead on the bolster for the entire time (or until you are ready to come out of the pose).

7. Precaution: If you are pregnant or have a hip or neck condition, consult your doctor before practicing this pose.

Uttanasana (Forward Fold) Bow-to-Grace with Two Chairs

1. Gather your props: two chairs, a mat, one block, two blankets, and one bolster.
2. Align the short edge of the mat against a wall, and place both chairs on the mat, one with its back against the wall for safety, and the other at least twelve inches from the first chair, seats facing each other.
3. On the seat of the second chair, stack the props as follows: the bolster horizontally, then one or both blankets, then the block horizontally at its lowest height.
4. Sit on the first chair, facing the second chair, feet planted, and draw the second chair closer to meet your knees.
5. Bow forward, as if in reverence, to rest your forehead on the rim of the block, and wrap your arms around the block, resting the forearms on the blanket.
6. Close your eyes, relax your entire body, and breathe into the pose for fifteen to twenty minutes (or until you are ready to come out of it). Feel your back body stretch and open.
7. Precaution: If you are pregnant, be sure there is room for your belly, or consult your doctor before practicing this pose.

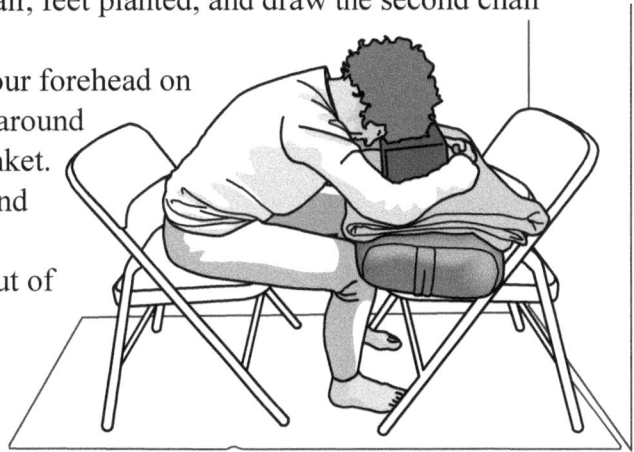

Viparita Karani (Legs Up the Wall) with Chair

1. Gather your props: a chair, a mat, two blankets, and an eyebag (optional).
2. Align the short edge of the mat against a wall, and place the chair on the mat, with its back against the wall for safety.
3. On the mat, facing the chair, and place a blanket where your head and neck will rest, folded thin enough to maintain the natural curvature of the neck.
4. Lie on the mat, placing your legs, at a 90-degree angle, on the seat of the chair. You may need to shift your buttocks closer to or farther from the chair. You might place a blanket on the chair for cushion or warmth.

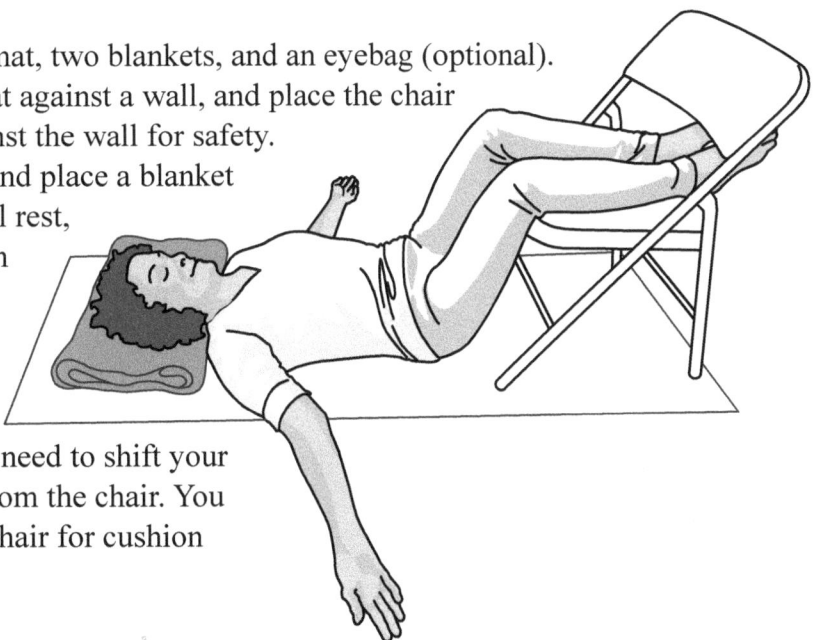

5. Bring your arms out to the side at a comfortable angle, palms up, or place your hands on your belly, fingers positioned in a mudra if you like. You might cover yourself with a blanket.

6. Close your eyes (or cover them with the eyebag), relax your entire body, and breathe into the pose for fifteen to twenty minutes (or until you are ready to come out of it). Feel the tension and fatigue release in your legs.

Supta Baddha Konasana (Bound Angle) Reclining

1. For options A and B, gather your props: a mat, four blocks, one bolster, four blankets, a yoga strap with a double-D ring, and an eyebag (optional).

2. From the top edge of the mat, position the bolster vertically, and place two blocks under the bolster as follows: the first, horizontally, at medium height, halfway up the bolster; the second, at the highest height, between the first block and the top of the bolster.

3. At the base of the bolster, place a blanket folded approximately two-feet-by-two-feet on the mat. Sit at the lower end of the bolster, on top of the blanket, tailbone just touching

OPTION A

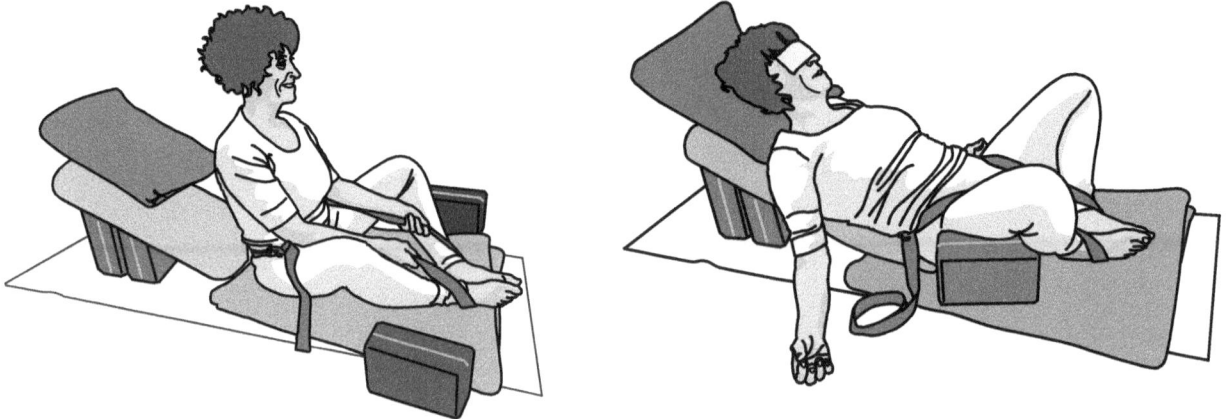

OPTION B

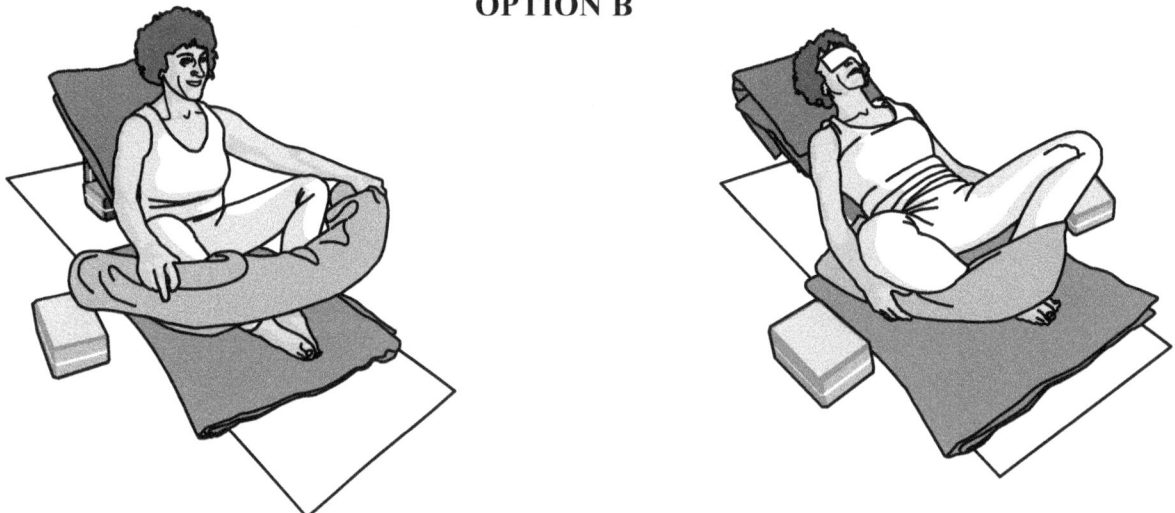

the bolster. Bend your knees, feet flat on the blanket, and slowly lie back on the bolster to make sure it supports you from sacrum to head.

4. Place a blanket on the bolster where your head and neck will rest, folded thin enough to maintain the natural curvature of the neck. Your forehead should be higher than your chin, your chin higher than your breastbone, and your breastbone higher than your pubic bone. Your torso should recline at a 45-degree angle to the floor.

5. Bring your soles together, allowing the knees to splay out. For option A, place a block under each outer thigh, at the height that feels better for your body. For option B, roll one of the blankets so that it's approximately four feet long and four to six inches wide, and wrap it around your ankles and under your shins, tucking the ends under the base of your hips.

6. For option A, make a big loop with the yoga strap, drop the loop over your head, and position it around your hips. Keeping your soles together, wrap a buckle-free part of the loop around your feet, and adjust the strap so that it runs low across your sacrum and over your inner thighs, and the tail of the strap is within easy reach.

7. For options A and B, slowly lie back on the bolster. For option A, tighten the strap just enough to hold your legs in place. You might position your fingers in a mudra and cover yourself with a blanket.

8. Close your eyes (or cover them with the eyebag), relax your entire body, and breathe into the pose for fifteen to twenty minutes (or until you are ready to come out of it). Feel your heart, abdomen, and pelvis open.

Babbling Mountain Brook

1. Gather your props: a mat, one bolster, three blankets, and an eyebag (optional).

2. On the mat, place a blanket where your head and neck will rest, folded thin enough to maintain the natural curvature of the neck.

3. Place a folded blanket where the center of your back will rest to maintain the natural curvature of the spine.

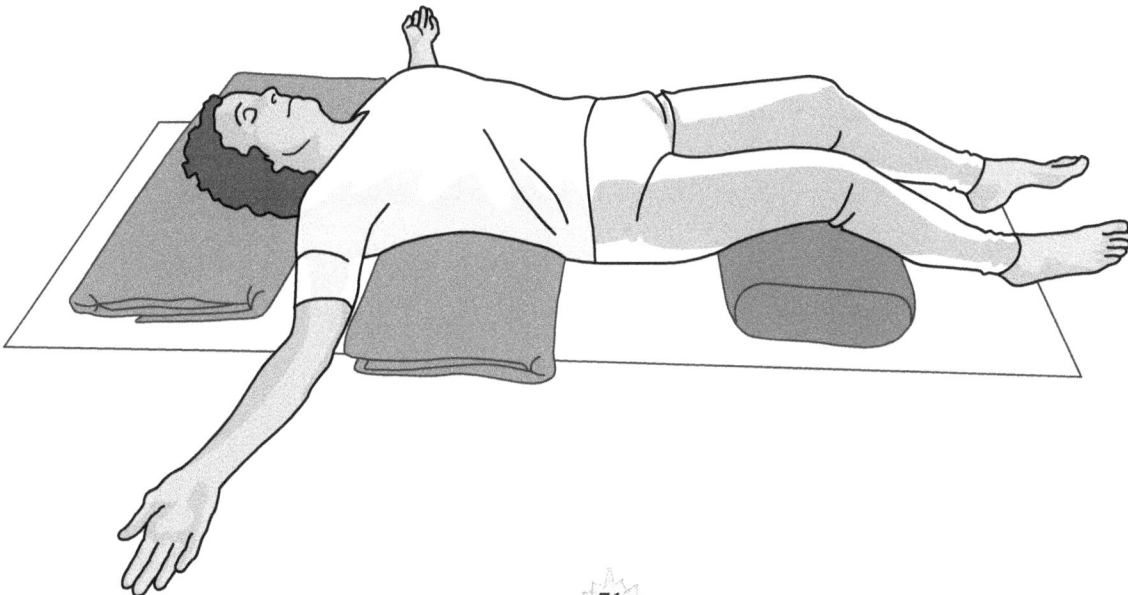

4. Lie on the mat, reposition the blankets as necessary, and place the bolster under your knees. You may need to refold the upper blanket so that the arch of your neck is completely supported: your head should gently tilt back; your throat should be open and relaxed.

5. Bring your arms out to the side, at a 90-degree angle, if possible, palms up, fingers positioned in a mudra if you like. You might cover yourself with a blanket.

6. Picture your body draped over the props like a wave. Envision a cool mountain brook flowing over stones.

7. Close your eyes (or cover them with the eyebag), relax your entire body, and breathe into the pose for fifteen to twenty minutes (or until you are ready to come out of it). Feel your throat, heart, and belly open.

8. Precaution: If you are pregnant or have high blood pressure or glaucoma, consult your doctor before practicing this inversion.

Anantasana (Sleeping Vishnu or Side-Lying Relaxation)

1. Gather your props: a mat, one bolster, four blankets, and an eyebag (optional).

2. On the mat, place a blanket folded to fit the mat's length and width.

3. On the blanketed mat, place a blanket where your head and neck will rest, folded thick or thin enough to maintain the natural curvature of your neck. Determine which side of your body you will lie on (left side is suggested if you are pregnant), and place a bolster and a rolled blanket at the side of the mat.

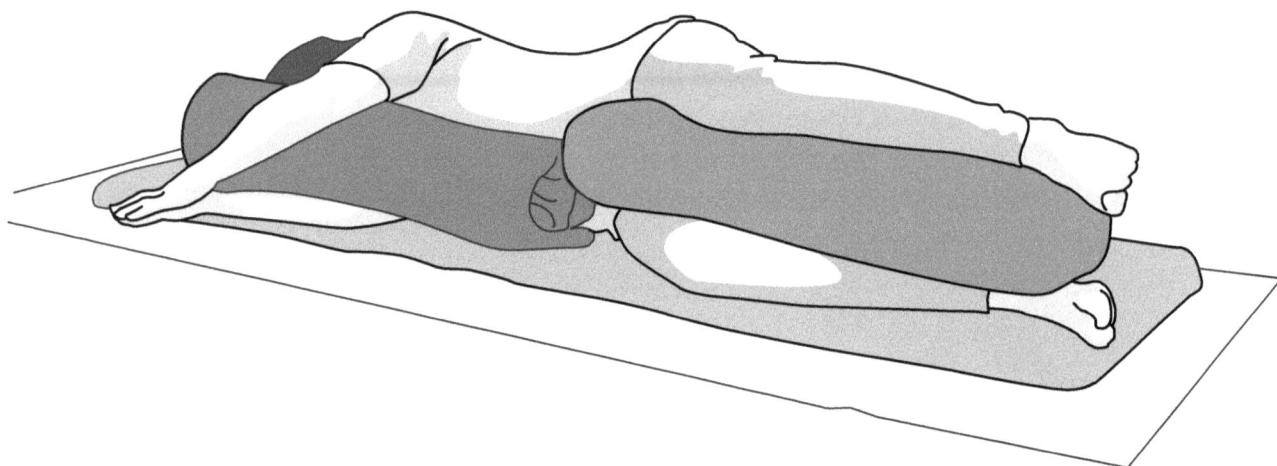

4. Lie on the mat on your preferred side, insert the bolster lengthwise between your knees and legs, and place a rolled blanket to hug to your front body. You might cover yourself with a blanket.

5. Close your eyes, relax your entire body, and breathe into the pose for fifteen to twenty minutes (or until you are ready to come out of it). Feel your body release tension as if it is preparing to sleep.

Setu Bandha Sarvangasana (Bridge)

1. Gather your props: a mat, one block, one bolster, two blankets, and an eyebag (optional).
2. Place the bolster vertically in the center of the mat, and lie on it so that your shoulders rest on the mat, just off the bolster.
3. Place the block, horizontally at its lowest height, under your ankles. If your head needs support, place a blanket under your head and neck, folded thin enough to maintain the natural curvature of the neck. You might cover yourself with a blanket.
4. Close your eyes (or cover them with the eyebag), relax your entire body, and breathe into the pose for fifteen to twenty minutes (or until you are ready to come out of it). Feel your heart center open as if a string attached to your chest is lifting it toward the ceiling.
5. To release the pose, engage the core, and bend the knees, one by one, to plant the feet on the mat, then roll to one side and sit up.
6. Precaution: If you are pregnant or have high blood pressure or glaucoma, consult your doctor before practicing this inversion.

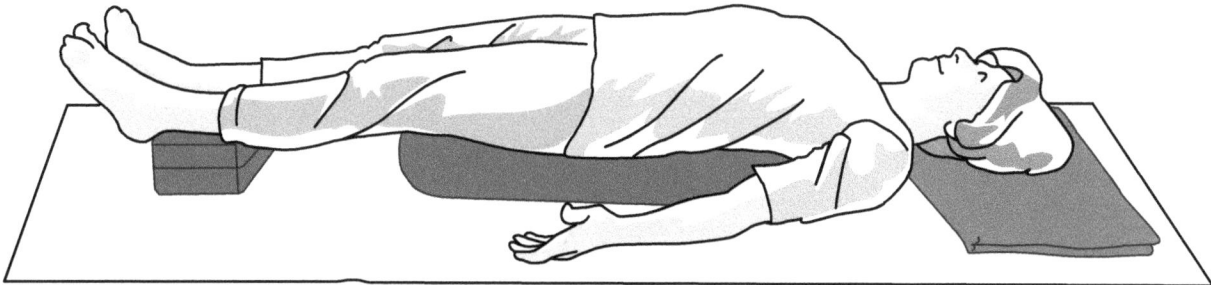

Restorative yoga truly restores the body, mind, heart, and soul by stimulating and soothing our organs. When we practice these passive poses with the support of props, the body and mind feel safe, grounded, and integrated—an act of self-care in this busy, noisy world. Sitting or lying down in silence for an extended period of time, honoring the body and the breath, takes exceptional patience, dedication, and courage.

Now let's close our practice with savasana, the final relaxation pose, also known as the "ultimate earth hug," the body securely planted on the ground.

Yoga is the innermost journey.
~Linda Anastasia Ransom

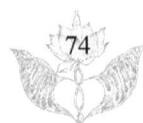

CHAPTER V

Final Relaxation: Savasana

Savasana, or *shavasana*, is the last pose of our yoga practice. In Sanskrit, *sava* means "corpse" and *asana* means "seat" or "posture," which is why savasana is also known as corpse pose. Savasana is considered a restorative pose, though it is held for five to fifteen minutes, and the head and heart are ideally aligned with each other.

Lying on a mat or resting in a chair may look easy, but savasana is considered the hardest pose in yoga because it is complete stillness. In this fast-paced world, we are challenged to surrender our "monkey mind," jumping from thought to thought like a monkey leaping from tree to tree. Alternatively, we may fall asleep in savasana, the essence of which is to remain relaxed with attention, to stay awake and aware in a resting position.

When we soften and close our eyes in savasana, our focus shifts to the movement of the breath, inhaling and exhaling. Nothing to do, think, feel, and nowhere to go. We connect with our most authentic self, the divine within. We have arrived into savasana.

Benefits:
- Calms the mind and central nervous system
- Stimulates the parasympathetic nervous system
- Relieves muscle tension and fatigue
- Lowers blood pressure and the metabolic rate
- Mitigate headaches, depression, anger, anxiety, and panic attacks
- Improves concentration, memory, and sleep quality
- Strengthens the immune and digestive systems
- Increases overall energy

Before coming into a savasana, be sure you have all your props, including an extra blanket to cover yourself once you're in the pose. To further stay warm, you might also wear socks and a sweater. To further relax, you might cover your eyes with an eyebag. Choose a pranayama—Ujjayi (p. 8) and Dirga (p. 9) are suggested—and a mudra (pp. 11–12) that matches the intention you may wish to focus the breath on.

After a session of yoga, the mind becomes tranquil and passive.
B.K.S. Iyengar, *Yoga: The Path to Holistic Health*[1]

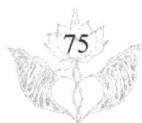

Traditional Savasana

1. Lie on your mat, flat on your back, feet slightly apart and arms at your sides, palms up.
2. Close your eyes, relax your entire body, and inhale and exhale slowly through your nose.
3. Continue for five to fifteen minutes (or until you are ready to come out).

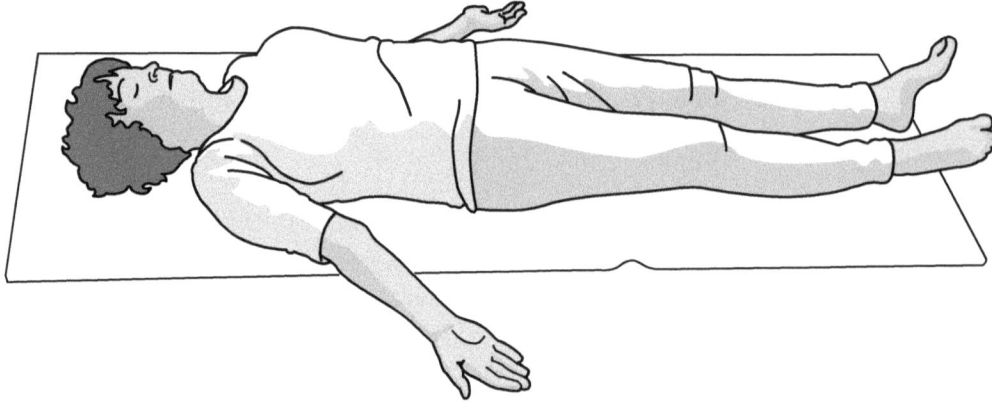

Cozy Lying-Down Savasana with Props

1. Gather your props: a mat, one bolster, three blankets, and an eyebag (optional).
2. On the mat, place a blanket folded to fit the mat's length and width.
3. On the blanketed mat, place a blanket where your head and neck will rest, folded thin enough to maintain the natural curvature of the neck.
4. Sit on the mat, place a bolster under your knees, and then lie flat on your back, feet slightly apart.
5. Bring your arms out to the side, at a 45-degree angle, palms up, fingers positioned in a mudra if you like. You might cover yourself with a blanket.
6. Close your eyes (or cover them with the eyebag), relax your entire body, and breathe into the pose for five to fifteen minutes (or until you are ready to come out of it).
7. Precaution: If you are pregnant or have high blood pressure or glaucoma, consult your doctor before practicing this pose.

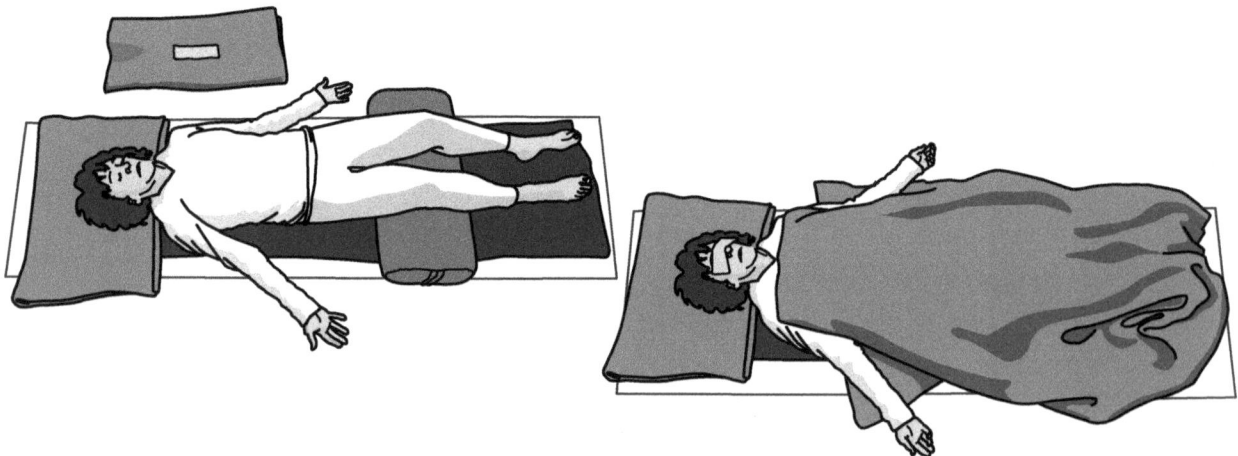

Viparita Karani (Legs Up the Wall) with Chair and a Touch of Heaven

1. Gather your props: a chair, a mat, one bolster, four blankets, and an eyebag (optional)
2. Align the short edge of the mat against a wall, and place the chair on the mat, with its back against the wall for safety.
3. Lie on the mat, facing the chair, and place three blankets as follows: one under your head and neck, folded thin enough to maintain the natural curvature of the neck; one folded approximately two-feet-by-two-feet under your back, from right below the shoulder blades to the sacrum; and one folded long enough to wrap around your legs from knees to toes.
4. Place your legs, at a 90-degree angle, on the seat of the chair. You may need to shift your buttocks closer to or farther from the chair. Wrap the blanket around your legs like a cocoon, place the bolster on top of your legs, and slowly lie back.
5. Bring your arms out to the side at a comfortable angle, palms up, or place your hands on your belly, fingers positioned in a mudra if you like. You might cover yourself with a blanket.
6. Close your eyes (or cover them with the eyebag), relax your entire body, and breathe into the pose for five to fifteen minutes (or until you are ready to come out of it).
7. To release the pose, remove the bolster, unwrap your legs, and, engaging the core, roll to one side and sit up.

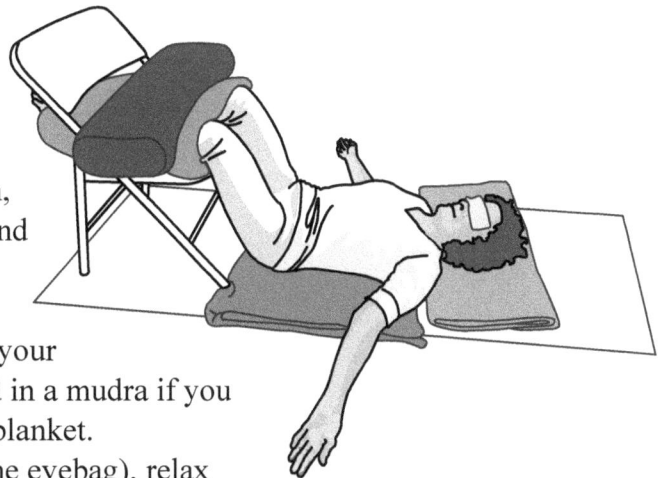

Bow-Your-Head Savasana

1. Gather your props: a chair, a mat, four blocks, and one bolster.
2. Place the chair on the mat, facing the other end of the mat.
3. Sit in the chair, feet parallel and hip-width apart on the floor. Place a block lengthwise under each foot.
4. Place the bolster horizontally across your thighs.
5. Stack one or two blocks on the bolster.
6. Bow your head to rest your forehead on the block(s).
7. Wrap your arms around the block(s).
8. Relax and breathe into the pose for five to fifteen minutes (or until you are ready to come out of it).

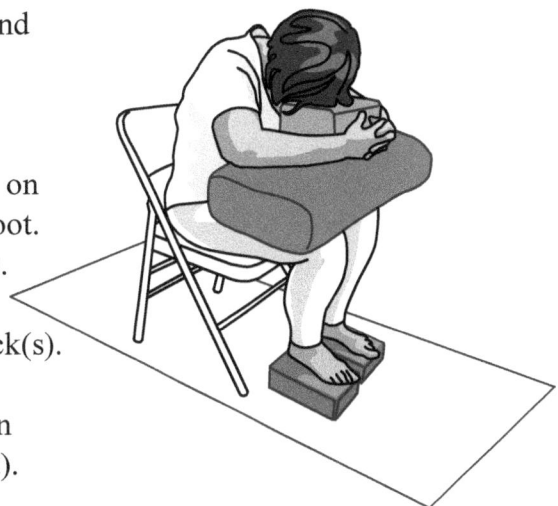

Blissful Savasana

1. Gather your props: a chair, a mat, three blocks, one bolster, and a yoga strap with a double-D ring.
2. Align the short edge of your mat against a wall, and place the chair on the mat, with its back against the wall for safety.
3. Sit in the chair, feet parallel and hip-width apart on the floor. Place a block lengthwise under each foot and vertically between your knees.
4. Loop the strap around your legs, about four inches above the knees, and tighten the strap so that the block is held without inward pressure from your legs.
5. Place the bolster behind your head and shoulders. Lean back and close your eyes, palms up or down on your thighs, fingers positioned in a mudra if you like.
6. Relax your entire body, and breathe into the pose for five to fifteen minutes (or until you are ready to come out of it).

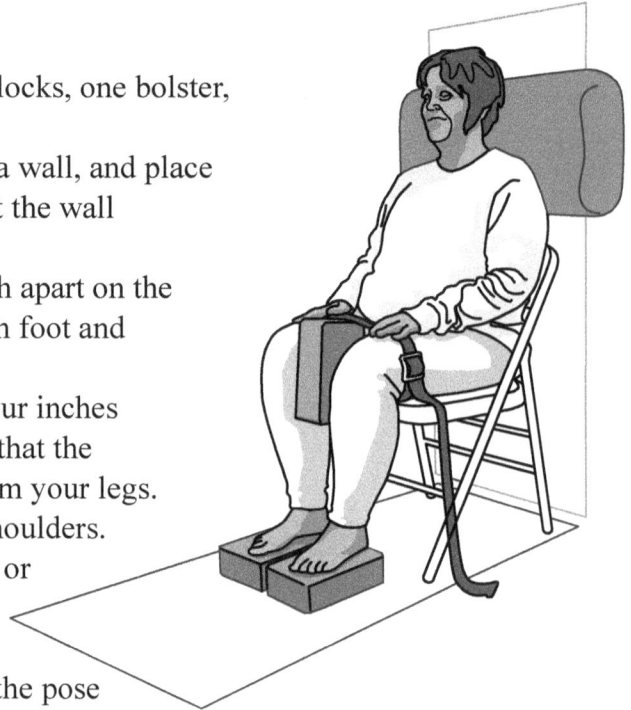

Mink-Stole Savasana

1. Gather your props: a chair, a mat, one block, one bolster, one blanket, and a yoga strap with a double-D ring.
2. Place the chair on the mat, facing the other end of the mat.
3. Sit in the chair, feet parallel and hip-width apart on the floor. Place the block vertically between your knees.
4. Loop the strap around your legs, about four inches above the knees, and tighten the strap so that the block is held without inward pressure from your legs.
5. Wrap a blanket around your neck, folded wide enough to support the head. The ends of the blanket should come approximately to your waist, evenly on both sides.
6. Place the bolster horizontally on the mat so that, when you extend your legs, your knees are slightly bent and the backs of your ankles rest on the front edge of the bolster. Your body may naturally recline about 105 degrees.

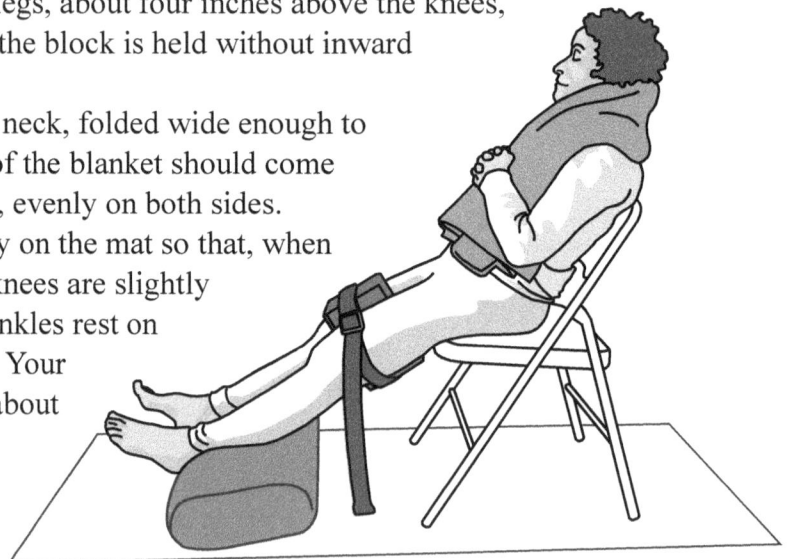

7. Wrap your arms around the blanket, clasping your hands.
8. Close your eyes, relax your entire body, and breathe into the pose for five to fifteen minutes (or until you are ready to come out of it).

Closing Your Practice

1. Position your body:
    a. Chair: Release your final savasana, place any props on the floor, and sit in Tadasana alignment.
    b. Mat: Release your final savasana, move any props to the side of the mat, and gently roll to one side into fetal position.
2. Pause for three Ujjayi breaths (p. 8).
3. If you are on a mat, slowly raise your body to a comfortable seated position.
4. Bring your hands to Anjali Mudra (p. 11) and bow your head.
5. Optional: Select a meditation (pp. 15–18).
6. Optional: Repeat the "Om" Mantra (p. 13) three times.
7. With head bowed, say aloud or silently, "Namaste. The light in me honors the light in you."
8. Thank your body, mind, and soul for all its good efforts.

Savasana, considered the master relaxation pose, is the concluding asana for nearly all yoga practices. What's noteworthy is that *savasana* is the first Sanskrit word learned by most yoga students. The resolve of savasana is to let go in order to purify the mind, body, and soul for a flourishing, sustainable life. Namaste, yogis. The light in me honors the light in you.

Coming up next are sample practice sequences for you to implement into your daily life. My wish for all the readers is to create your own yoga lesson plans and set up a daily practice or at least three days a week of yoga, pranayama, and meditation. Perhaps some days your practice will be filled with more asanas, or your well-being may desire more restoratives or meditation. Design your practice to nourish your body, mind and soul. Whatever you choose to do, do it with intention and pure love. Your life will change forever!

---

1. B.K.S. Iyengar, *Yoga: The Path to Holistic Health* (New York: DK Publishing, 2008), p. 37.

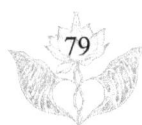

Yoga is the essence of being.
~Linda Anastasia Ransom

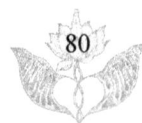

CHAPTER VI

Healing Chair Yoga Sequences

Ready to design your own Healing Chair Yoga class? For your convenience, this chapter presents four sample sequences to practice and to model your own sequences on. Two are a total-body sequence; the third is a restorative sequence, each running approximately one hour, shorter or longer depending on how long you hold the poses; and the fourth is a thirty-minute total-body sequence for when you're short on time. Following the four samples are template instructions for designing your own sixty- and thirty-minute sequences. (For a fifty-minute Healing Chair Yoga sequence, see this video: https://www.youtube.com/watch?v=SdaSdwIMnjw.)

Be sure to read through the previous chapters, asana by asana, before practicing these sequences.

Sample Sequence #1: Total Body (60-min)

Gather all the props needed for the asanas below and have them close by for easy access.

Alignment

Tadasana (Mountain Pose) (p. 5)

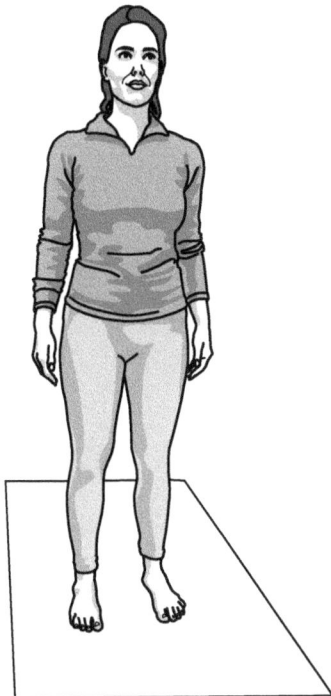

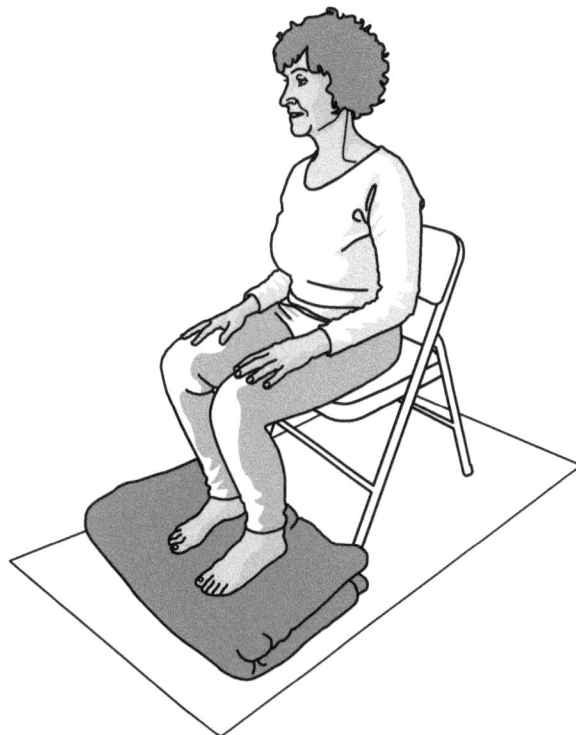

Pranayama

Observing the Breath and Setting an Intention (p. 7)
Ujjayi Pranayama (p. 8)
Optional: Gyan Mudra (p. 11)
Optional: "Om" Mantra (p. 13)

Foot Openers

Foot Massage (p. 22)

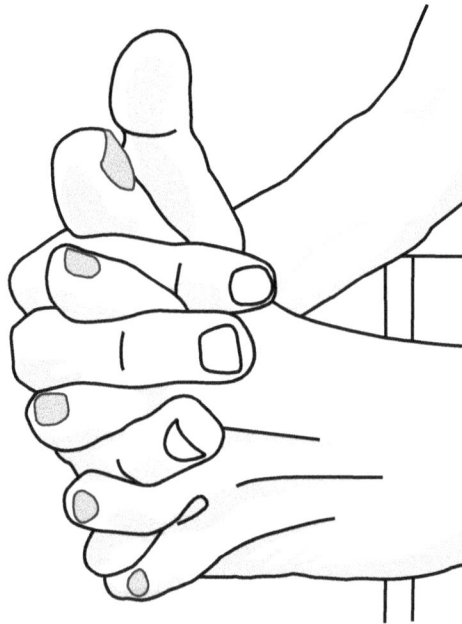

Arch Stretch II (p. 23)

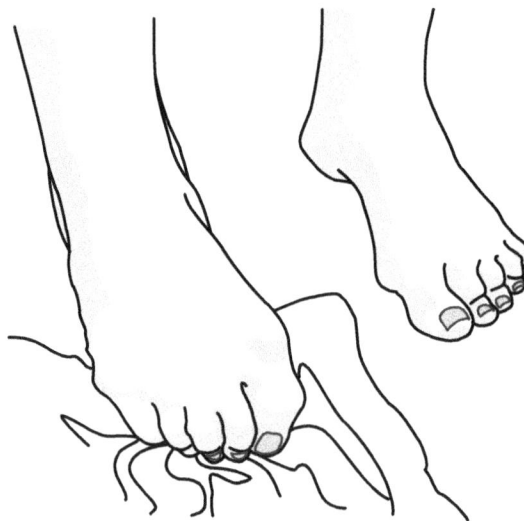

Wrist, Hand, and Finger Openers

Karate-Kid Hands Sprinkling Fairy Dust (p. 29)

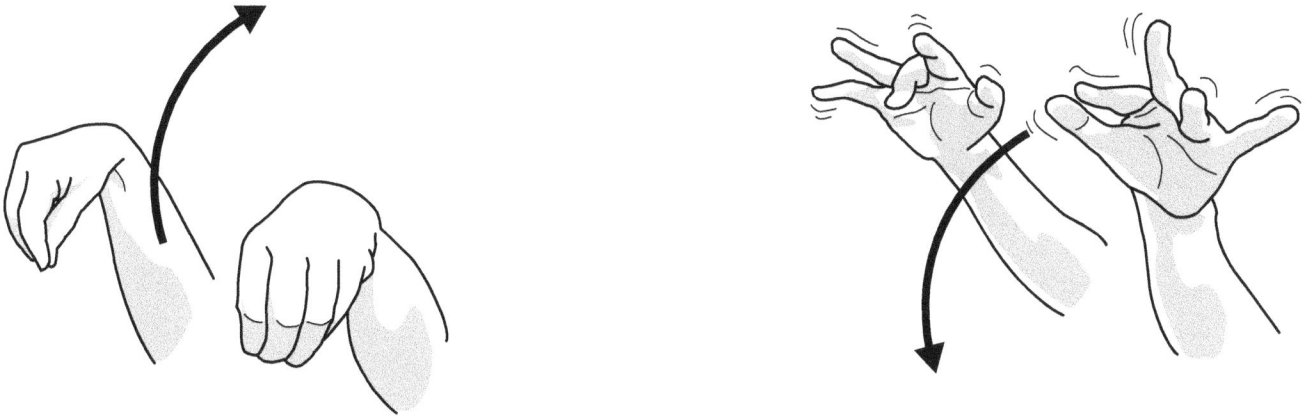

Figure Eights (p. 31)

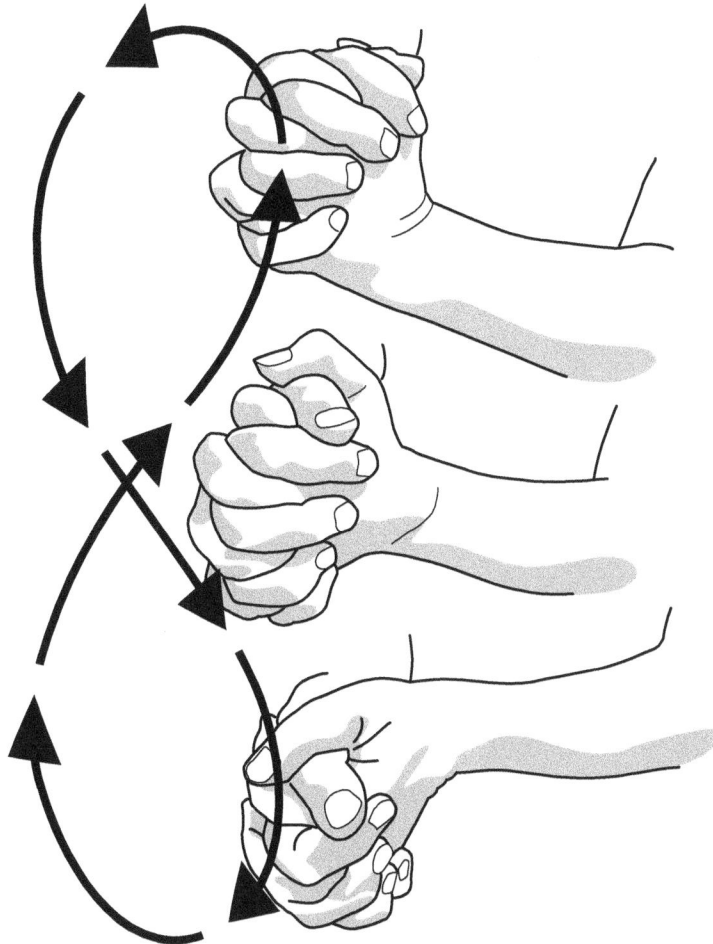

Shoulder and Neck Openers

Garudasana (Eagle Arms) (p. 37)

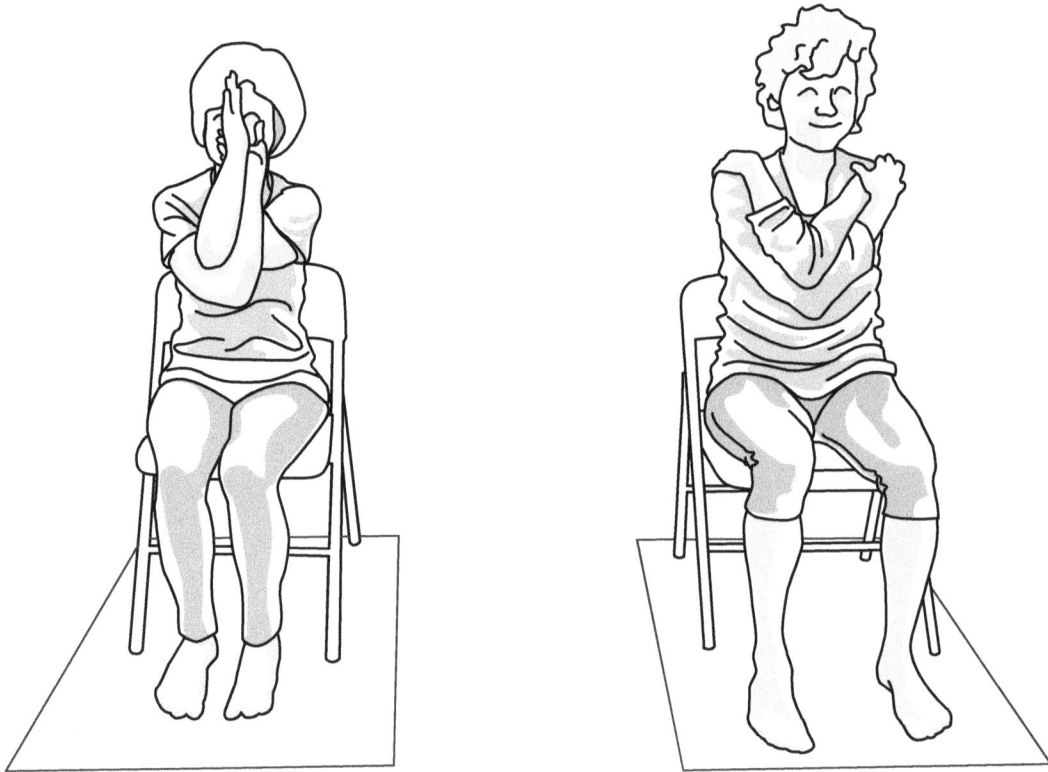

Shoulder Opening with Strap (pp. 38–39)

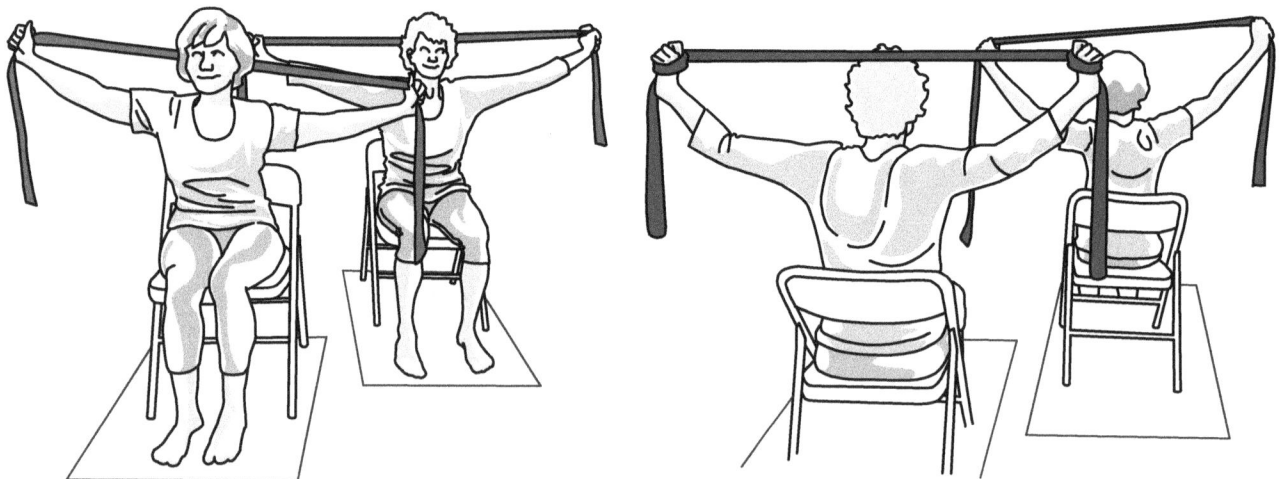

Heart Openers

Grounding Heart Meditation (pp. 41–42)

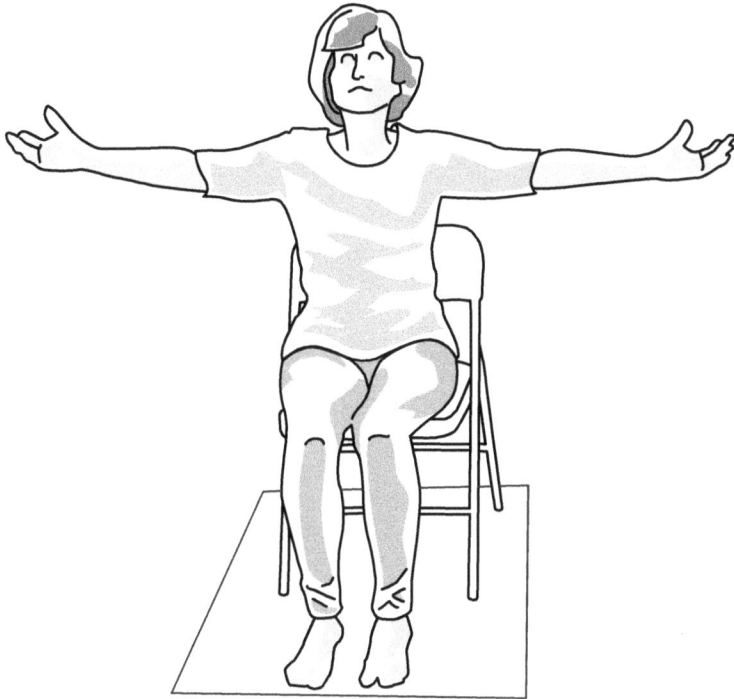

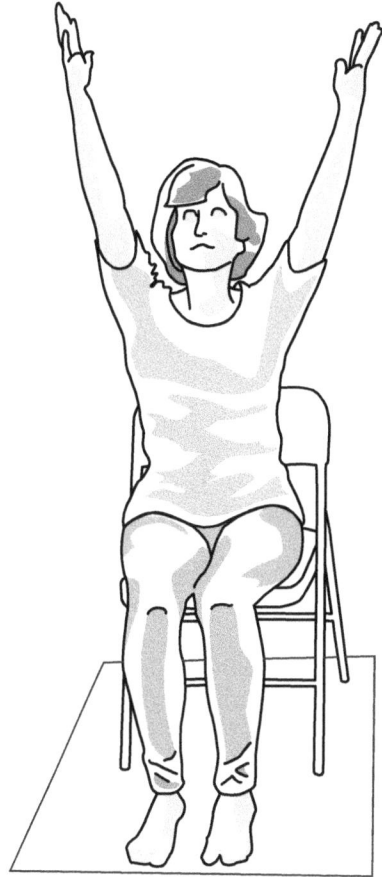

Cat-Cow Flow (pp. 42–43)

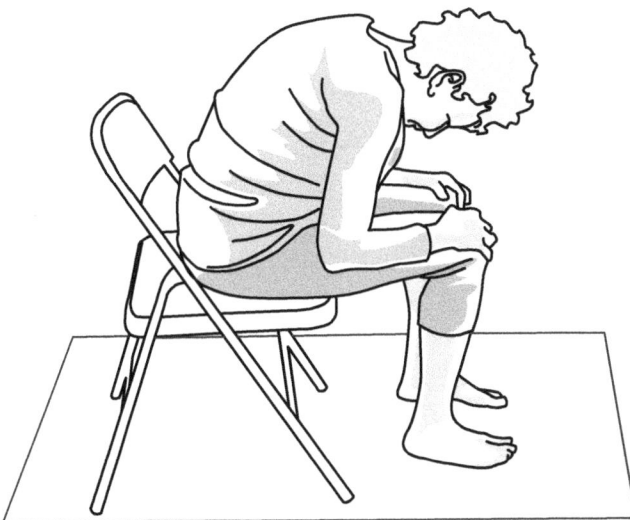

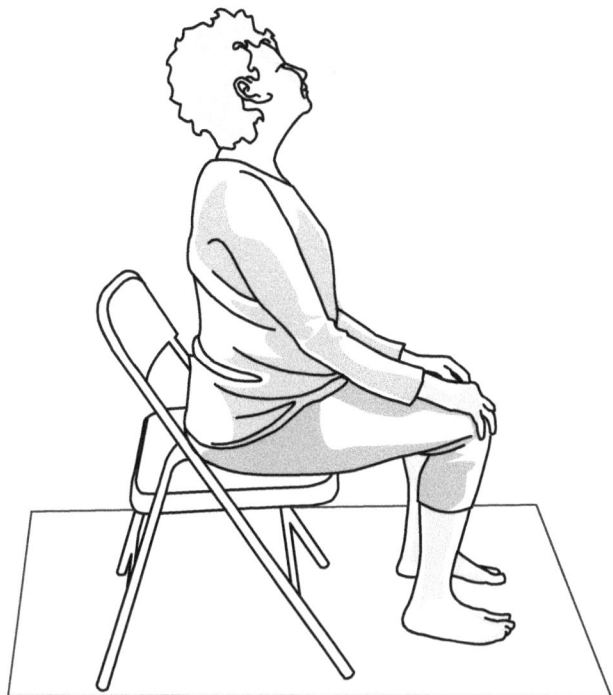

Twists

Vakrasana (Twist) Seated (p. 47)

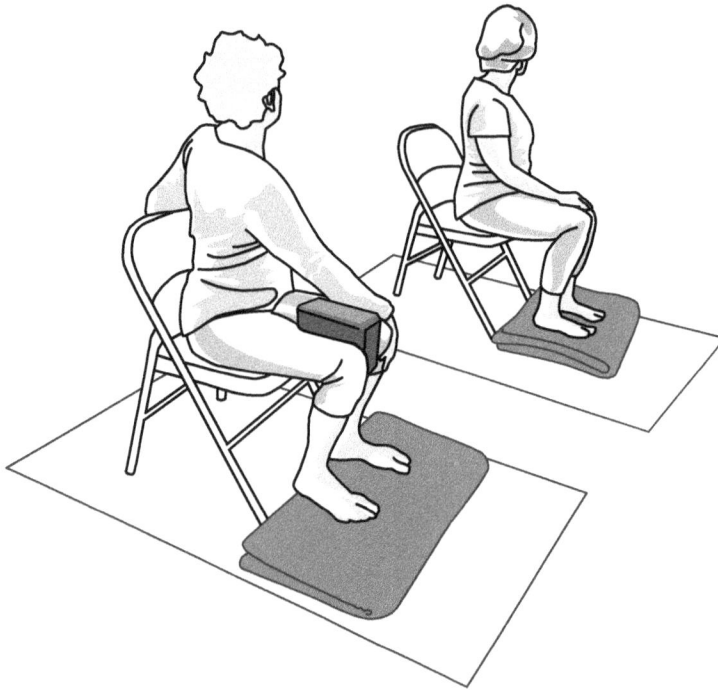

Side-Body Opening (p. 47)

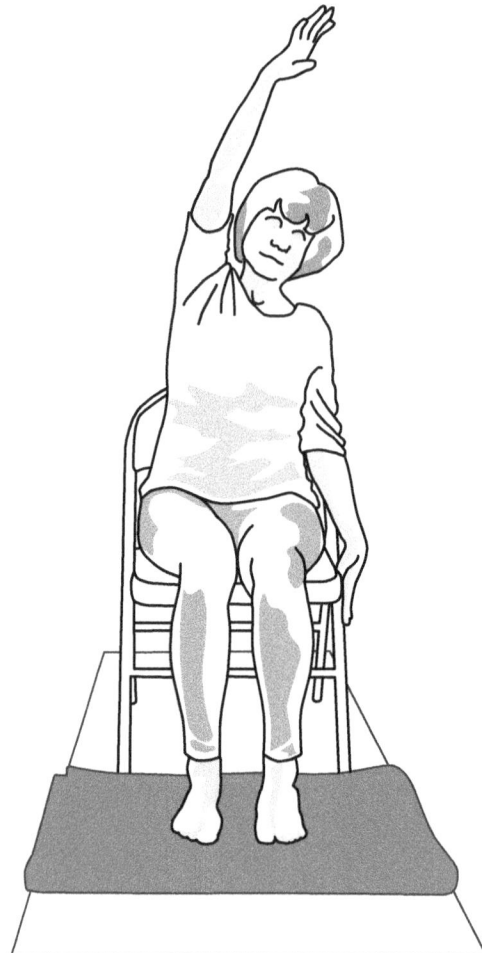

Hip Openers

Abductors and Adductors (pp. 50–51)

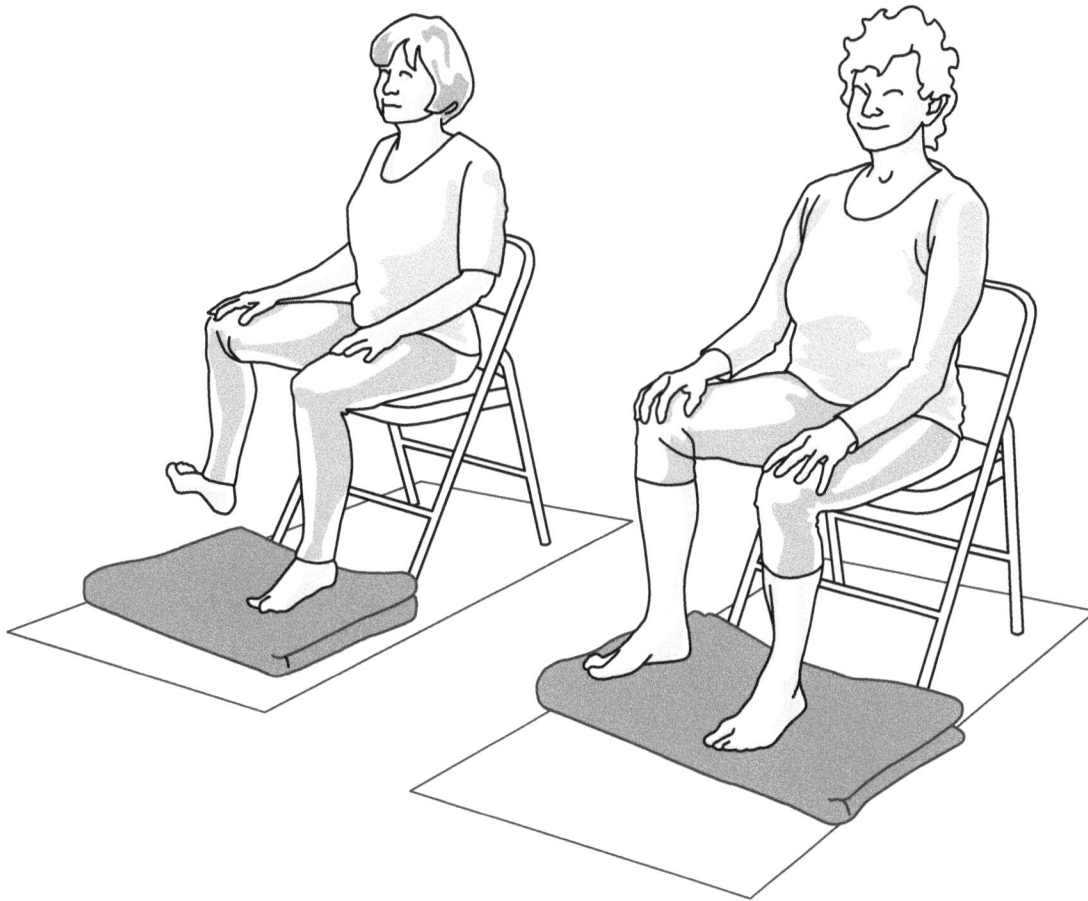

Kapotasana (Pigeon) (p. 52)

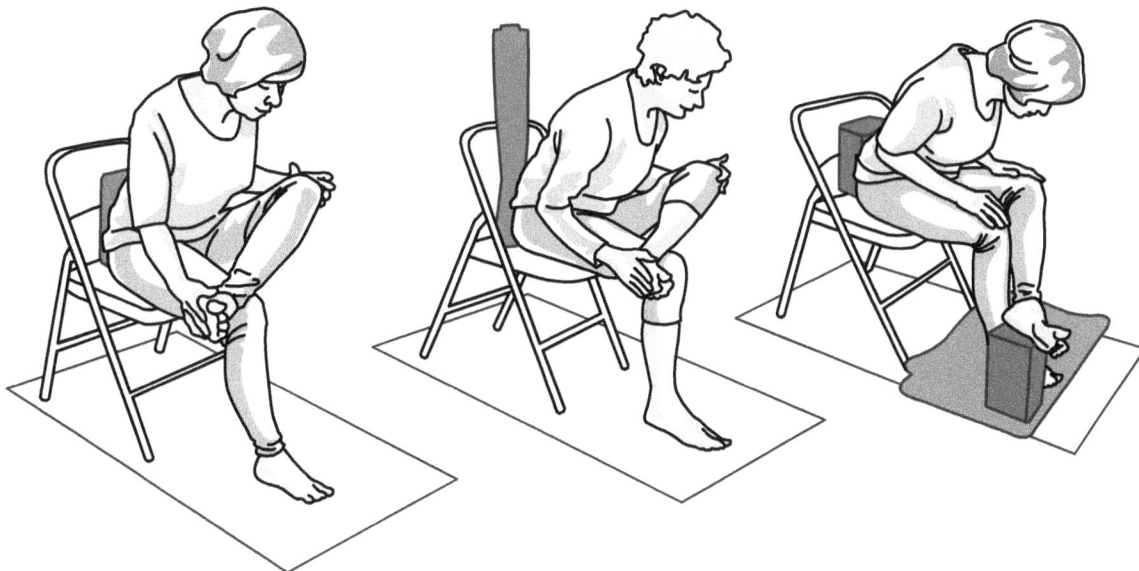

Balance

Vriksasana (Tree) (pp. 58–59)

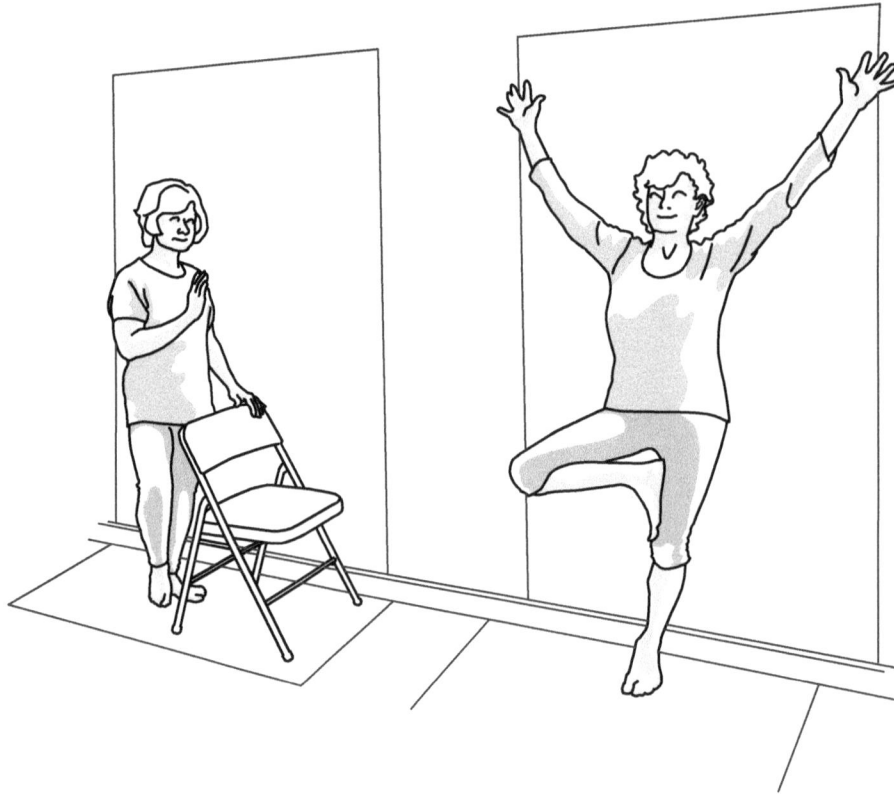

Virabhadrasana III (Warrior III) (p. 59)

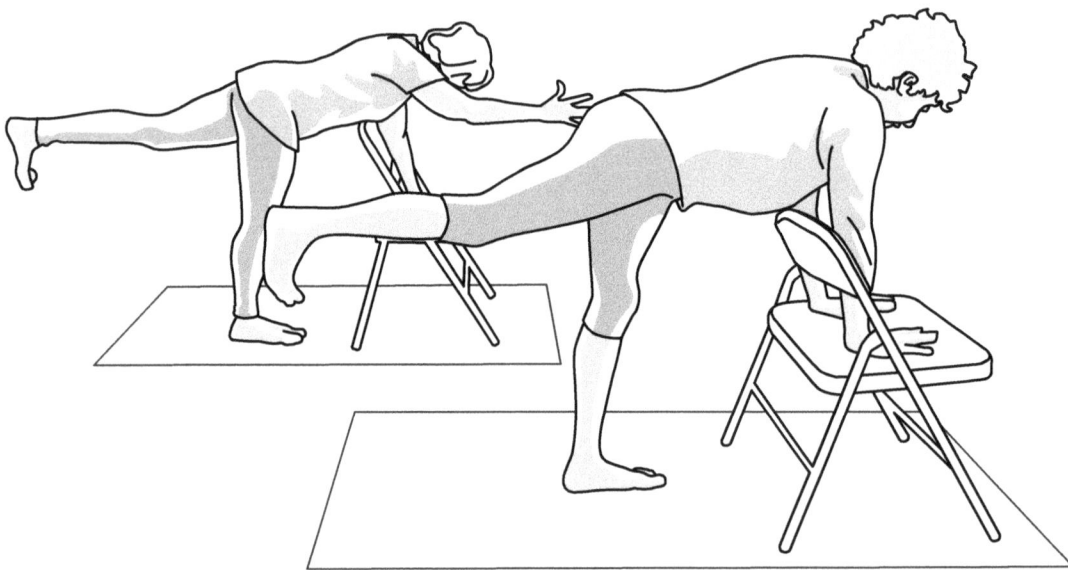

Restorative

Supta Baddha Konasana (Bound Angle) in Chair (p. 66)

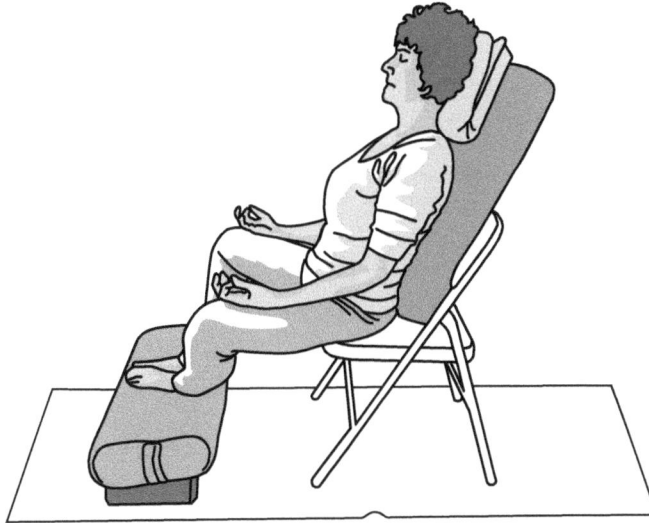

Savasana

Bow-Your-Head Savasana (p. 77)

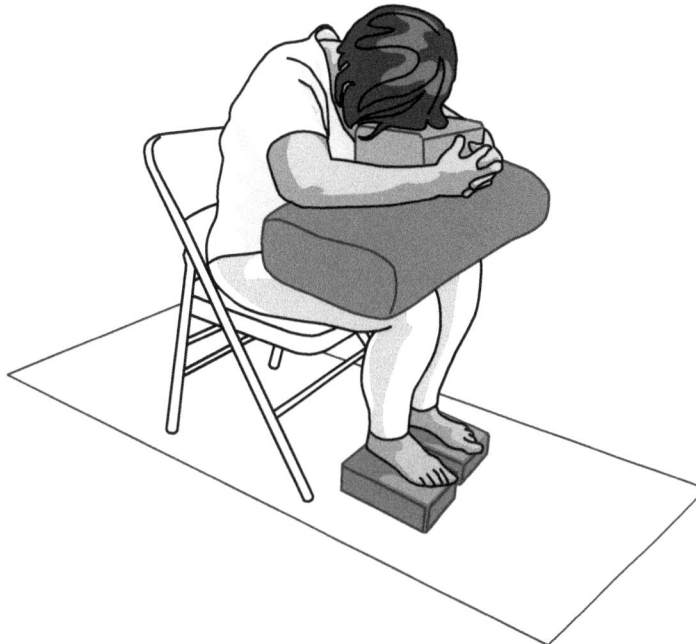

Closing Your Practice (p. 79)

Sample Sequence #2: Total Body (60-min)

Gather all the props needed for the asanas below and have them close by for easy access.

Alignment

Tadasana (Mountain Pose) (p. 5)

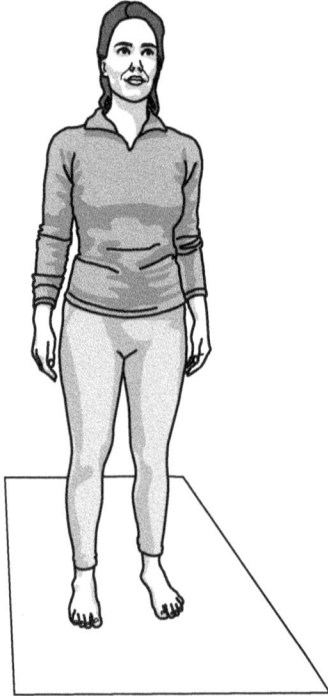

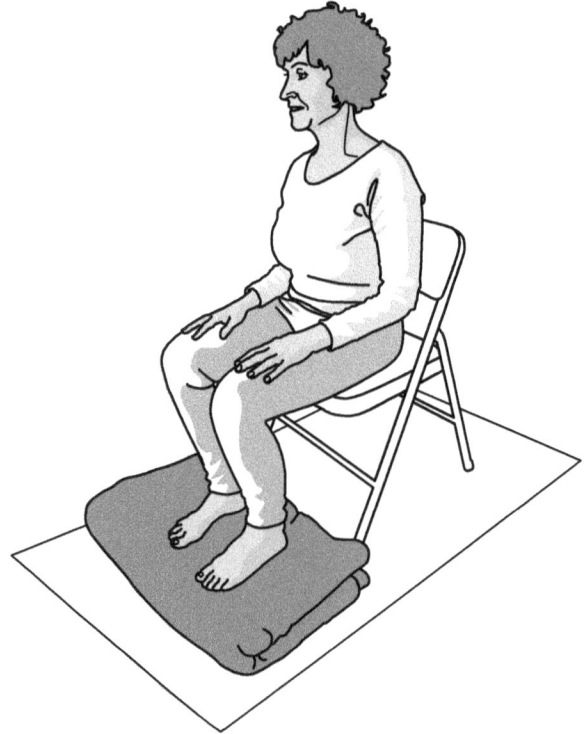

Pranayama

Observing the Breath and Setting an Intention (p. 7)
Sama Vritti Pranayama (p. 9)
Optional: Shuni Mudra (p. 12)
Optional: "All Is Well" Mantra (p. 13)

Foot Openers

Ball Massage (p. 24)

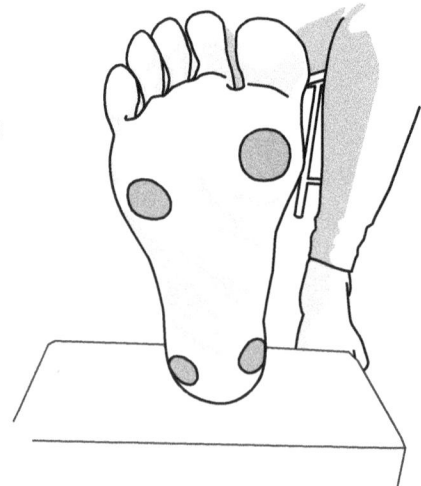

Virabhadrasana I (Warrior I), Back Heel Up and Down (p. 26)

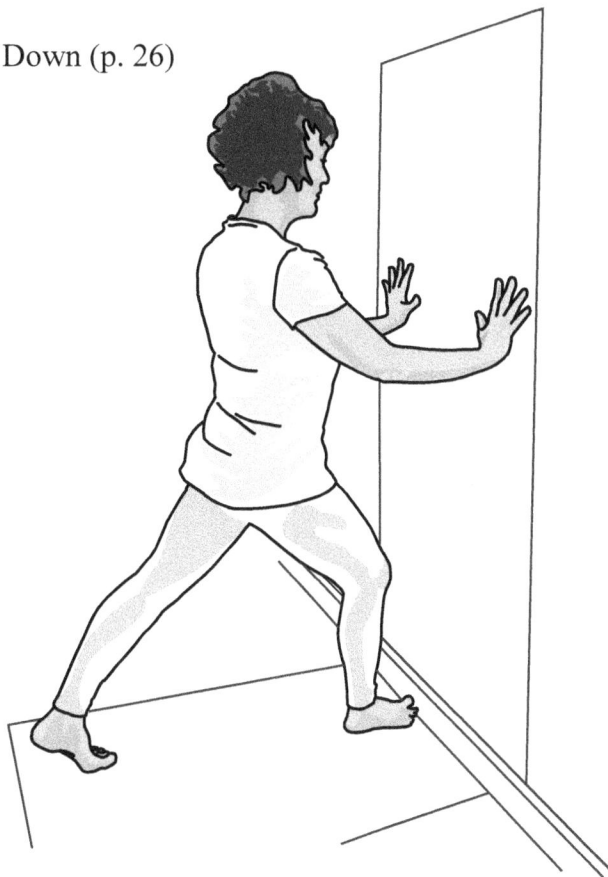

Wrist, Hand, and Finger Openers

Shake, Shake, Shake (p. 27)

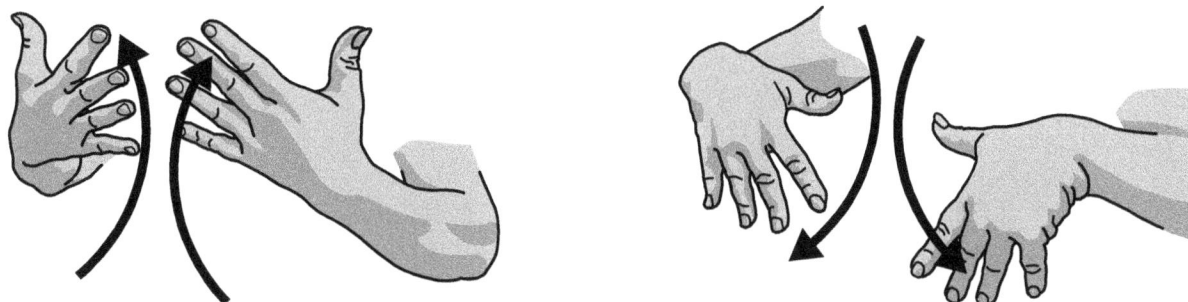

Palm Up (p. 28)

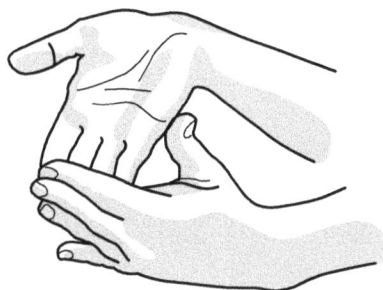

Shoulder and Neck Openers

Trapezius and Neck Stretch (p. 35)

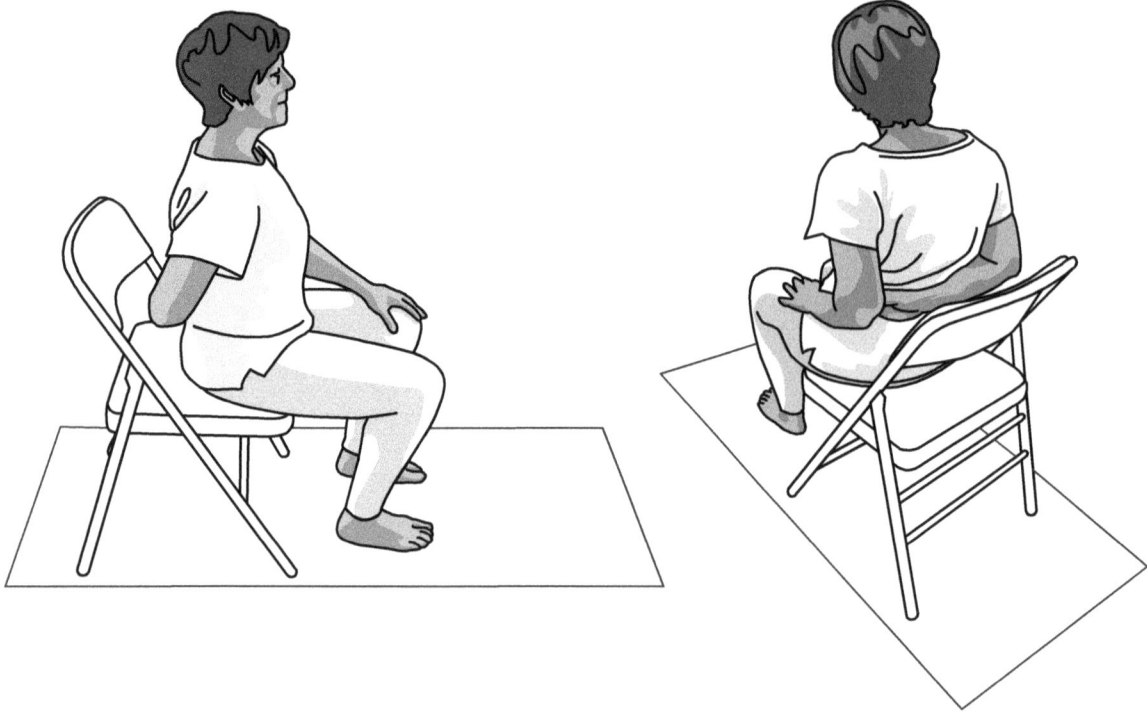

Earlobe Tug and Neck Stretch (p. 36)

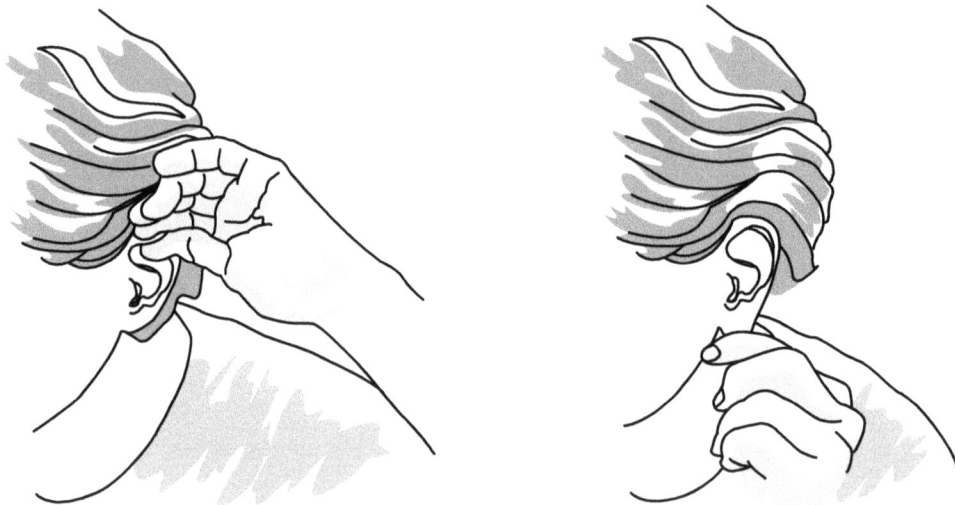

Heart Openers

Adho Mukha Svanasana (Downward-Facing Dog) to
Urdhva Mukha Svanasana (Upward-Facing Dog) (p. 44)

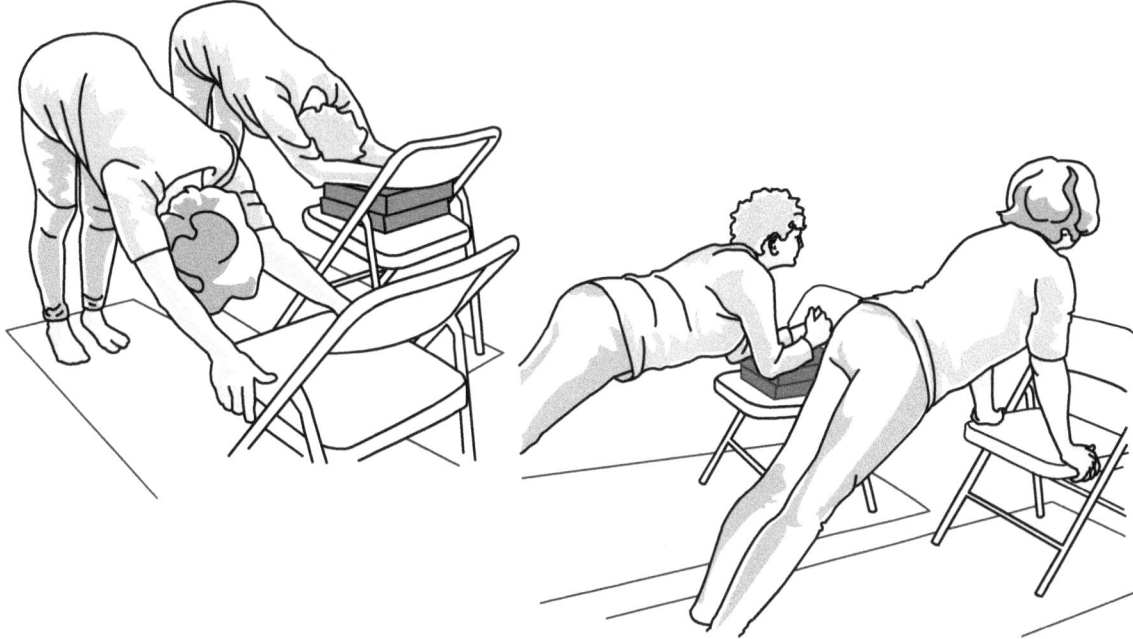

Virabhadrasana I (Warrior I) to Viparita Virabhadrasana (Reverse Warrior) Flow (p. 46)

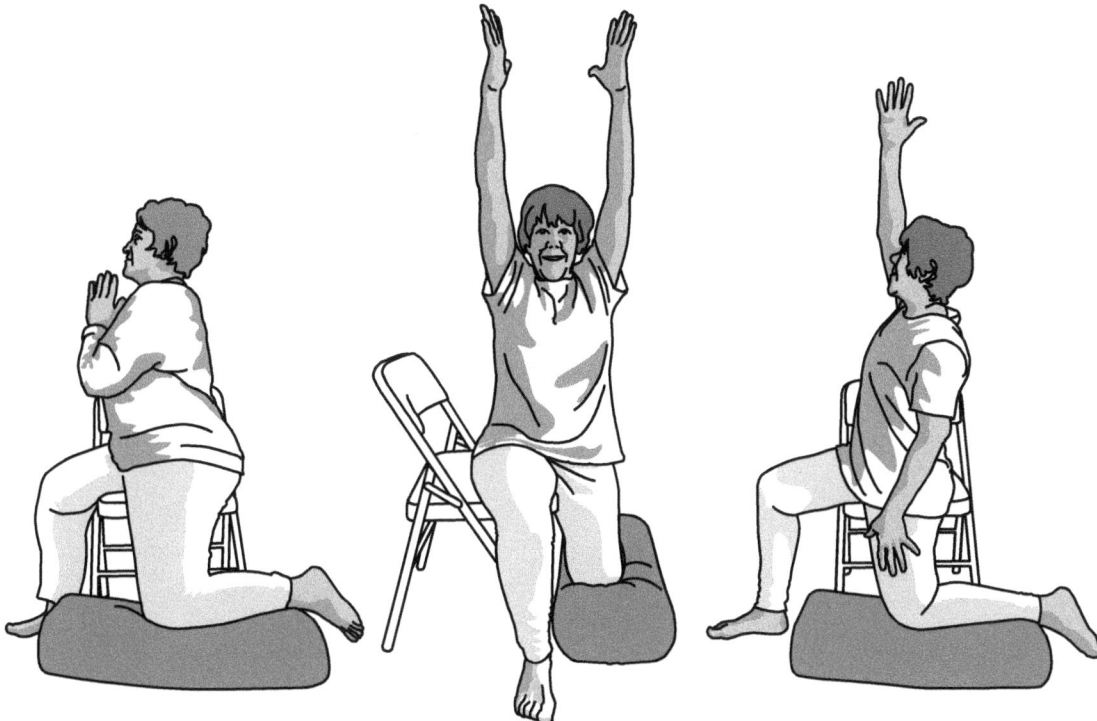

Twists

Vakrasana (Twist) Standing (p. 48)

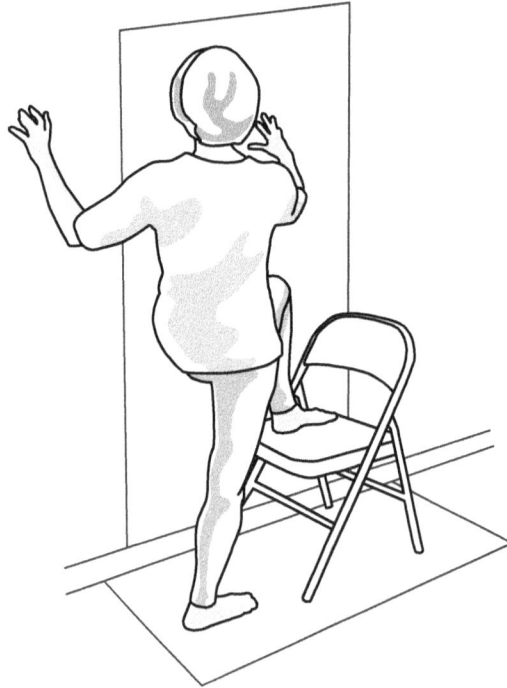

Vakrasana (Twist) Seated with Block (pp. 49–50)

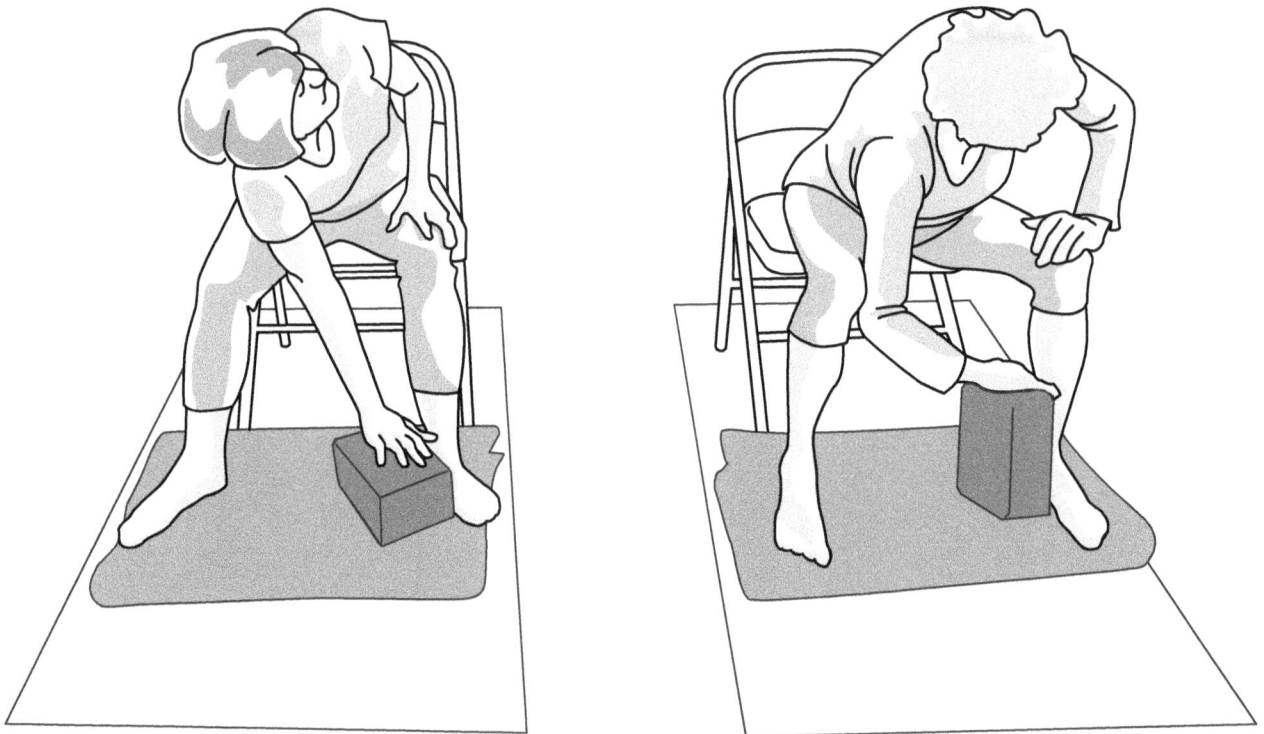

Hip Openers

Straight-Leg Abductor and Adductor (pp. 51–52)

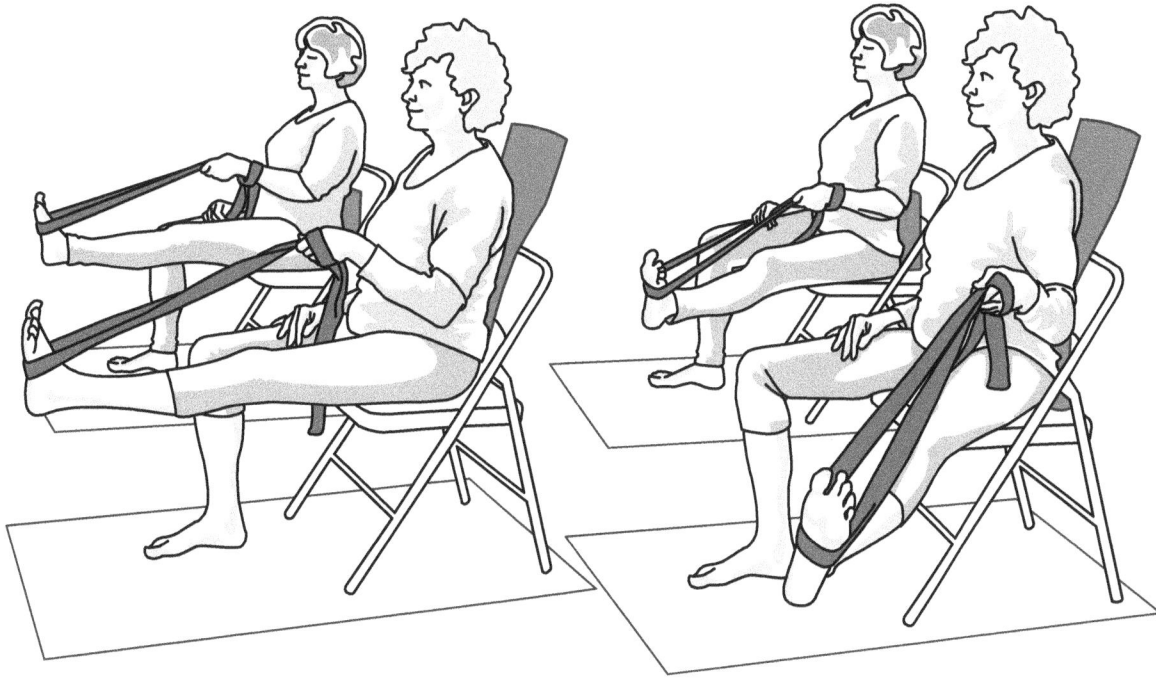

Virabhadrasana I (Warrior I) (p. 53)

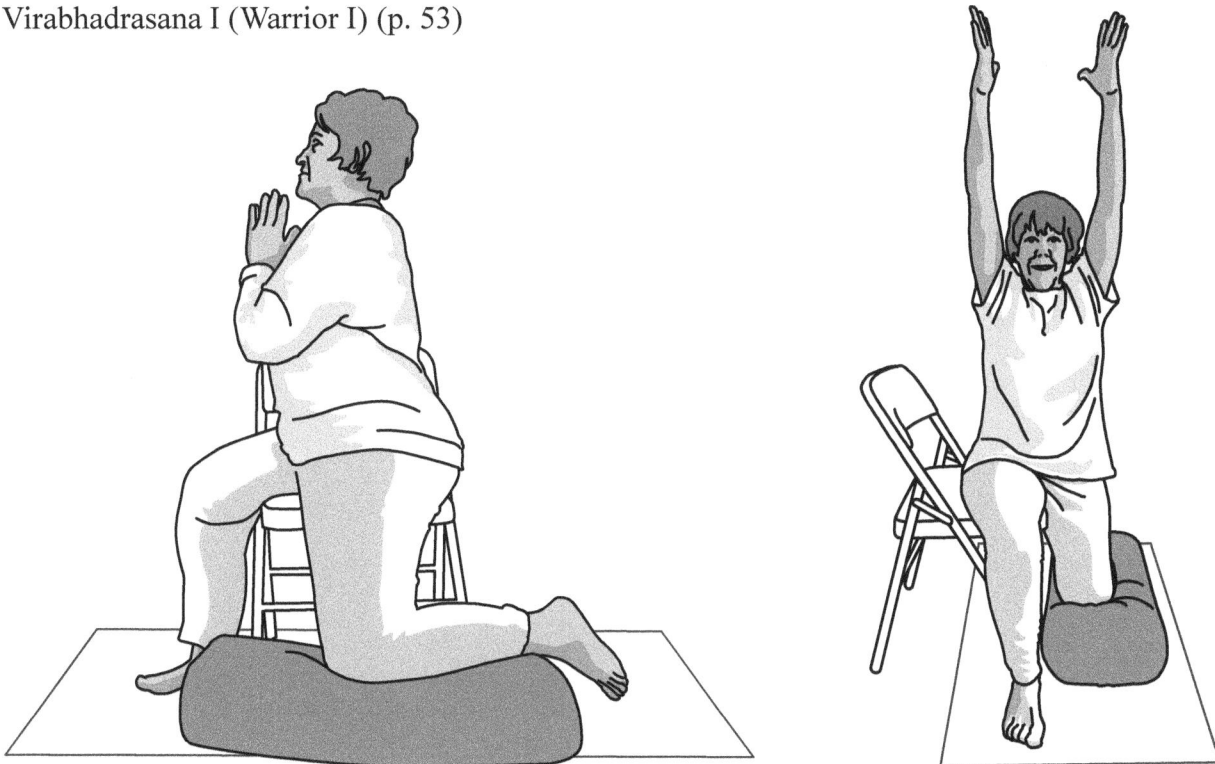

Balance

On Your Toes (p. 57)

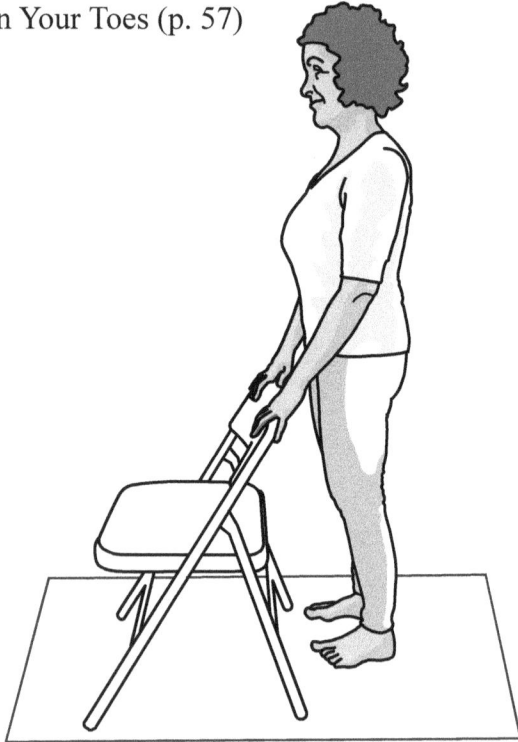

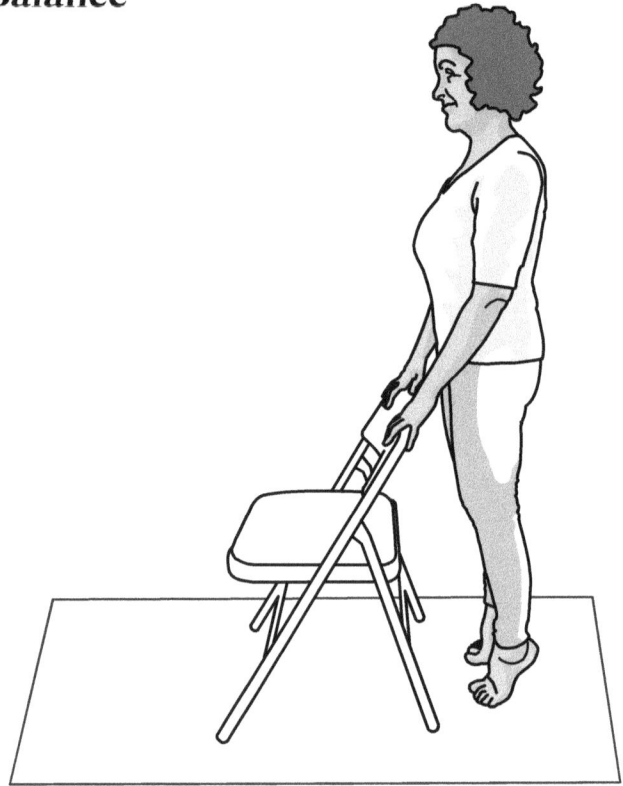

Ardha Chandrasana (Half Moon) (p. 60)

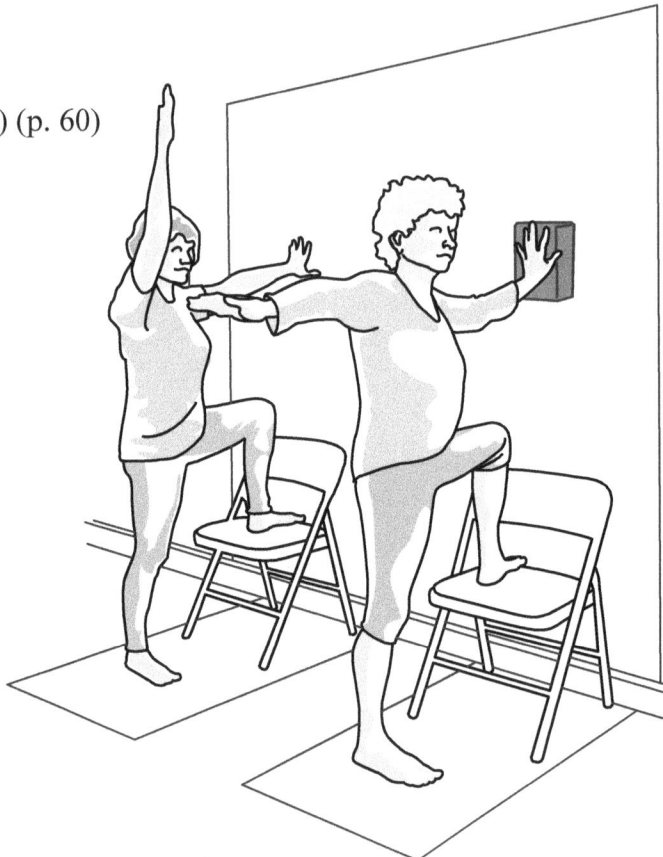

Restorative

Uttanasana (Forward Fold) Big Hug with Two Chairs (pp. 68–69)

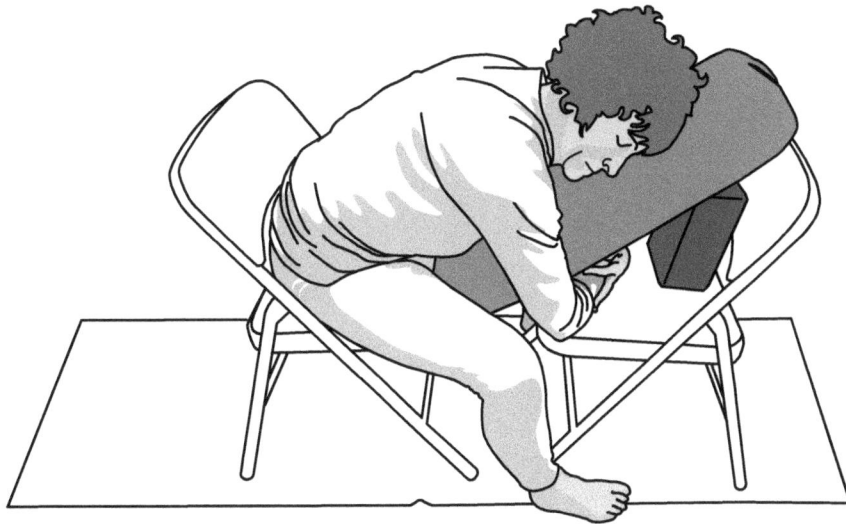

Savasana

Mink-Stole Savasana (pp. 78–79)

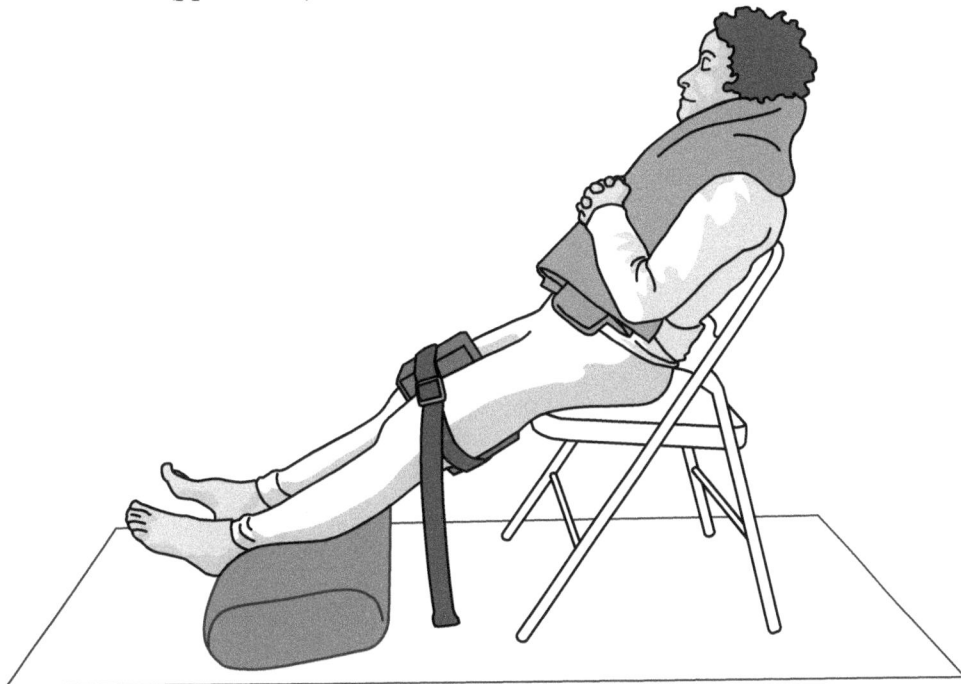

Closing Your Practice (p. 79)

Sample Sequence #3: Restorative (60-min)

Gather all the props needed for the asanas below and have them close by for easy access.

Alignment

Tadasana (Mountain Pose) (p. 5)

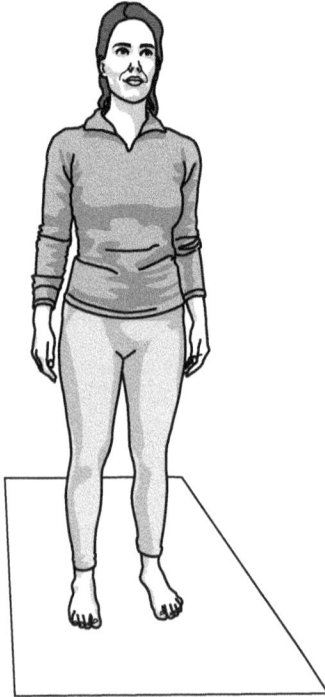

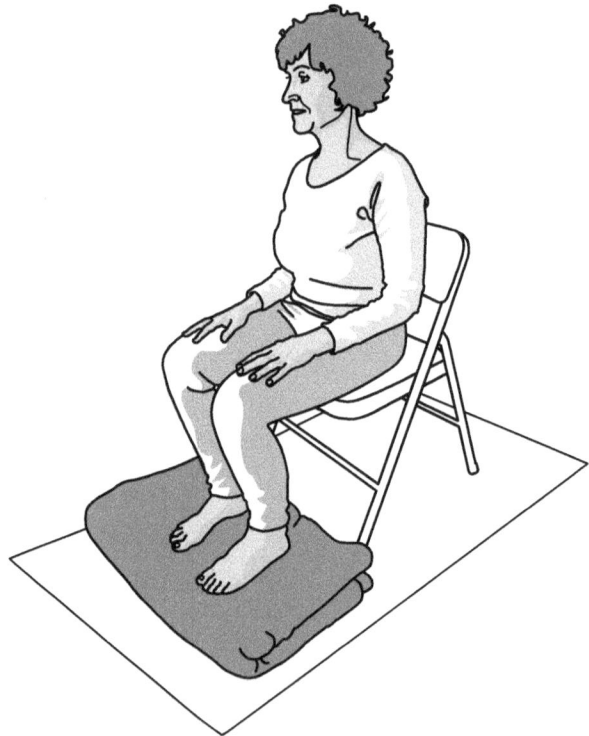

Pranayama

Observing the Breath and Setting an Intention (p. 7)
Dirga Pranayama (p. 9)
Optional: Buddhi Mudra (p. 12)
Optional: "Sat Chit Ananda" Mantra (p. 13)

Restorative

Supta Baddha Konasana
(Bound Angle) in Chair (p. 66)

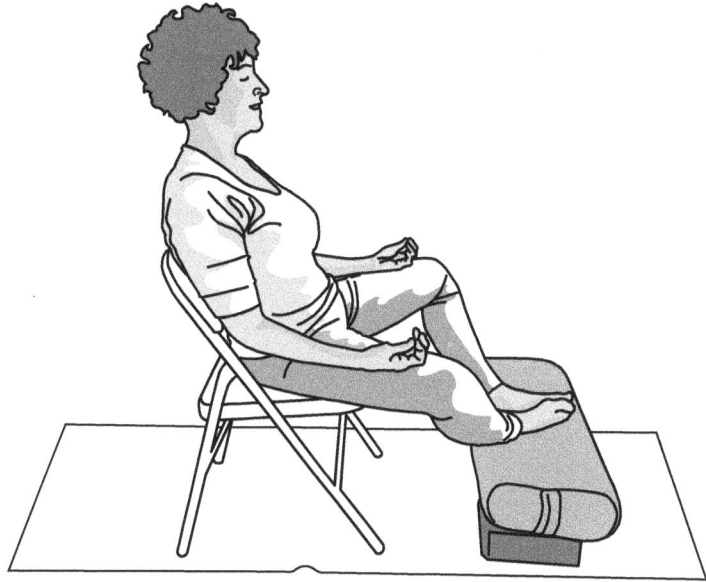

Uttanasana (Forward Fold) Big Hug with Two Chairs (pp. 68–69)

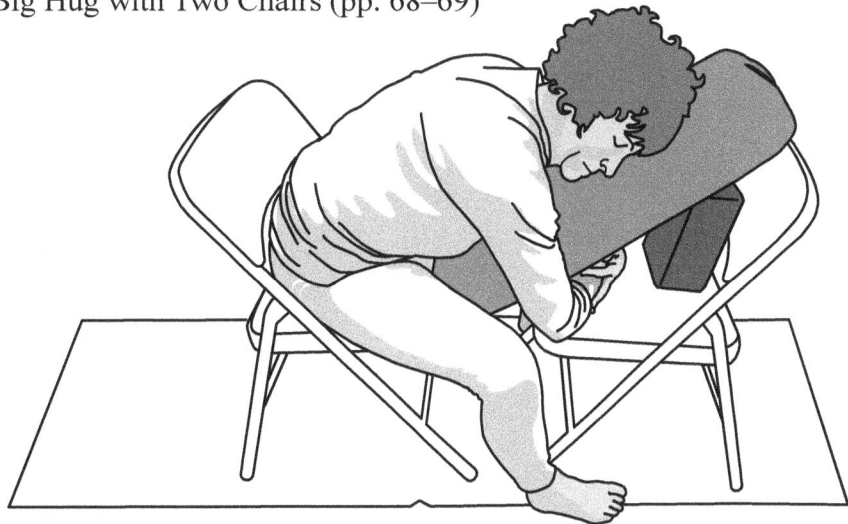

Anantasana (Sleeping Vishnu or Side-Lying Relaxation) (p. 72)

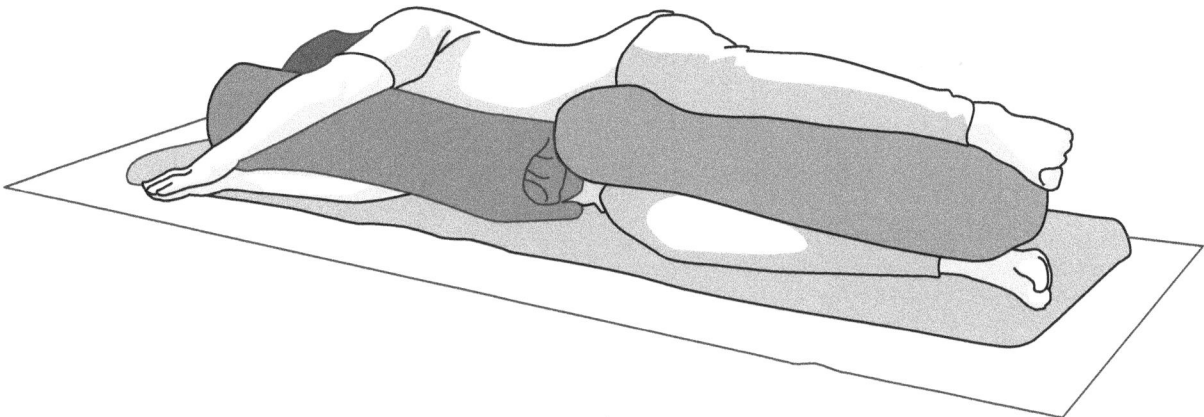

Savasana

Viparita Karani (Legs Up the Wall) with Chair and a Touch of Heaven (p. 77)

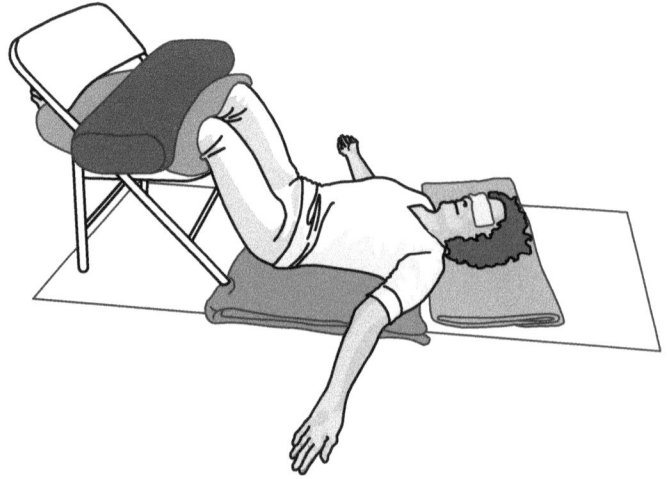

Closing Your Practice (p. 79)

Sample Sequence #4: Total Body (30-min)

Alignment

Tadasana (Mountain Pose) (p. 5)

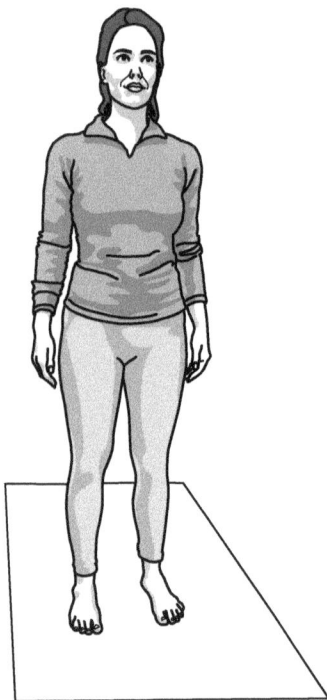

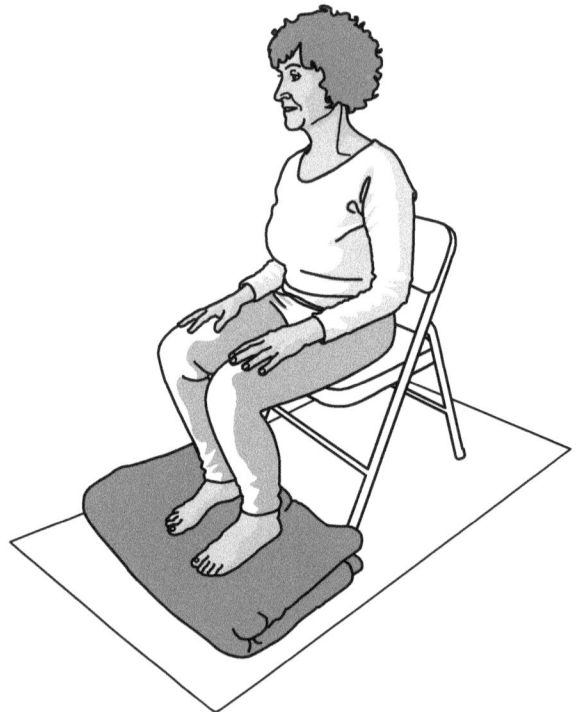

Pranayama

Observing the Breath and Setting an Intention (p. 7)
Ujjayi Pranayama (p. 8)
Optional: Gyan Mudra (p. 11)
Optional: "Om" Mantra (p. 13)

Foot Opener

Flex, Point, Floint (p. 23)

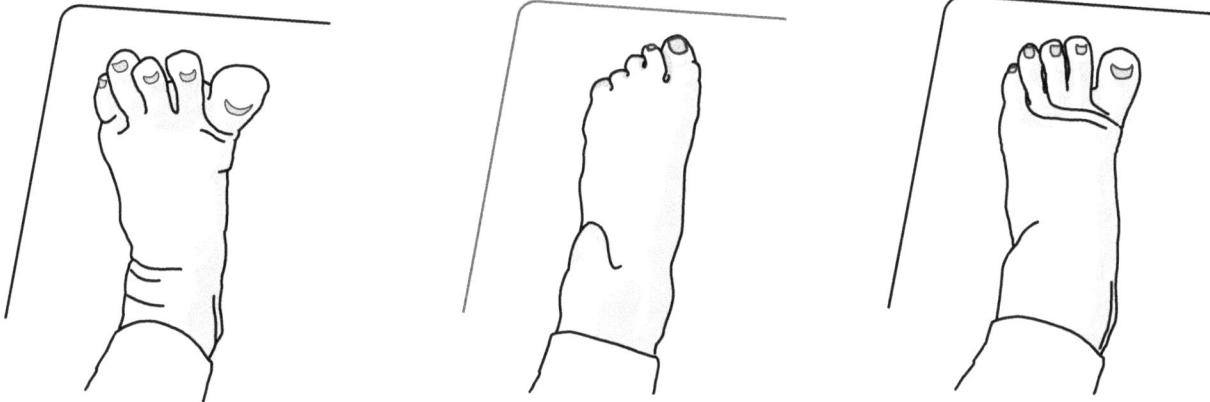

Wrist, Hand, and Finger Opener

Karate-Kid Hands Sprinkling Fairy Dust (p. 29)

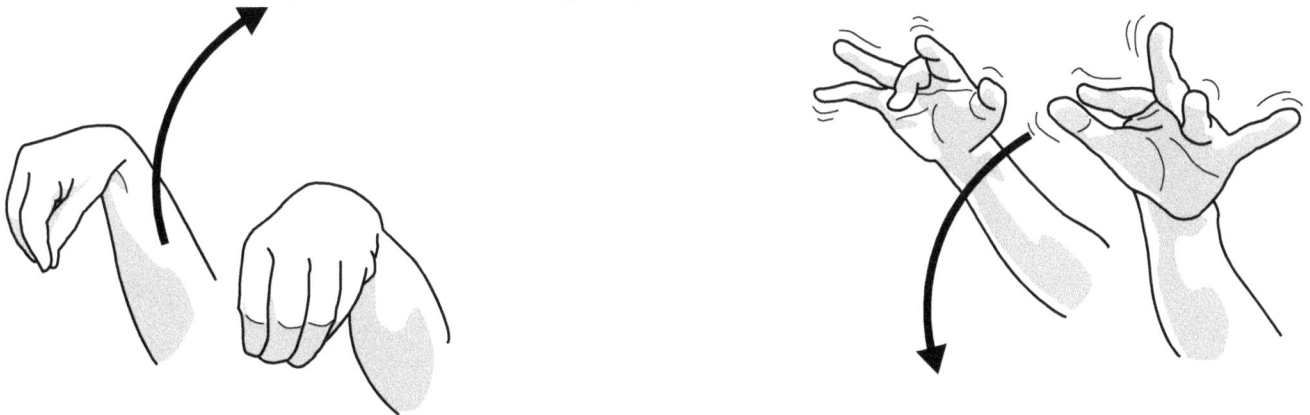

Shoulder and Neck Opener

Clock at the Wall (pp. 40–41)

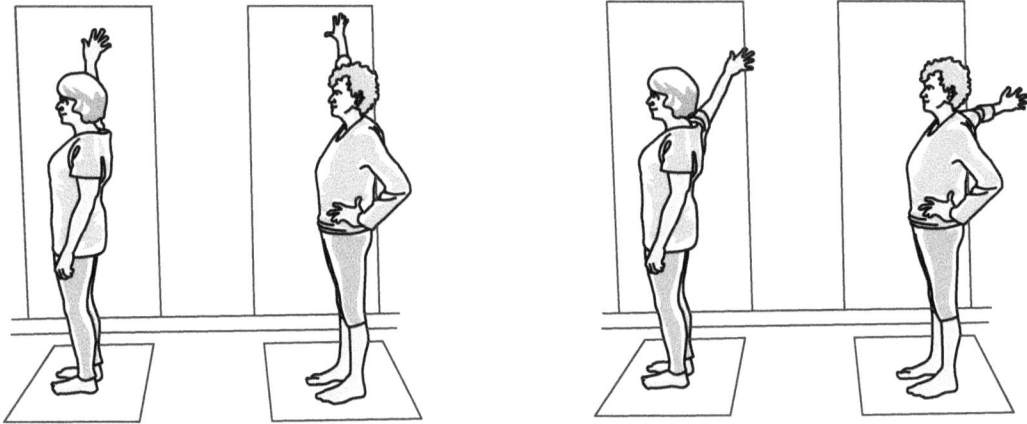

Heart Opener

Salamba Setu Banda Sarvangasana (Bridge) (pp. 43–44)

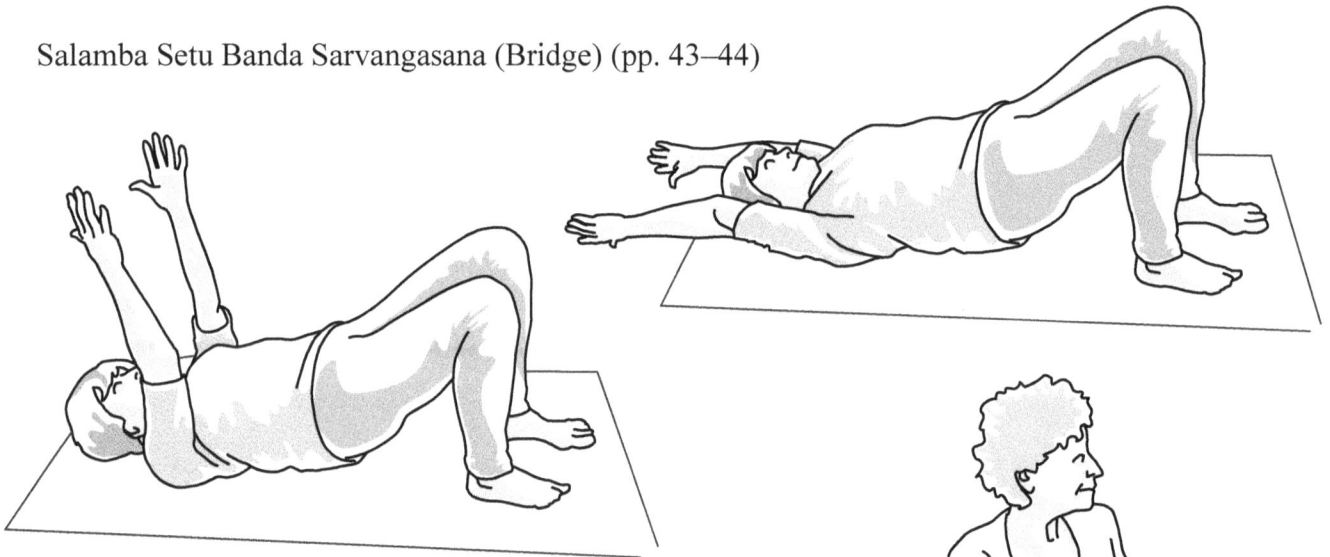

Twist

Vakrasana (Twist) Side-Saddle (p. 48)

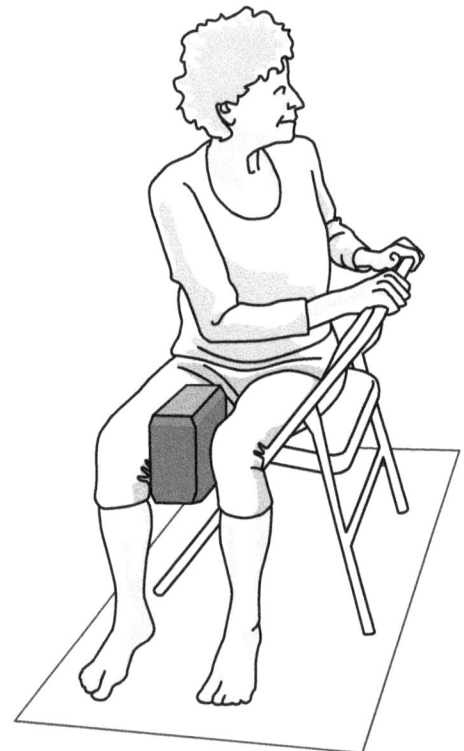

Hip Opener

Knee Circles (p. 53)

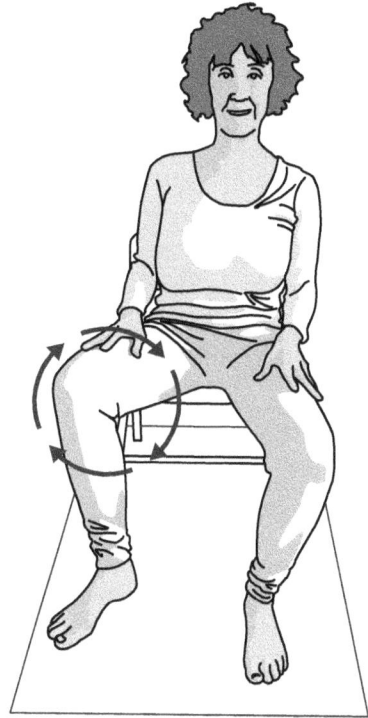

Balance

Natarajasana (Dancer) (pp. 62–63)

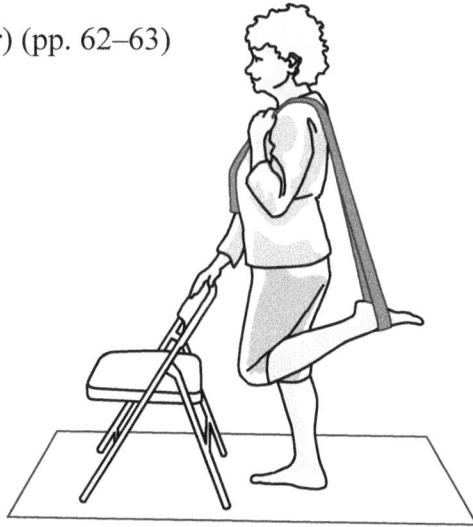

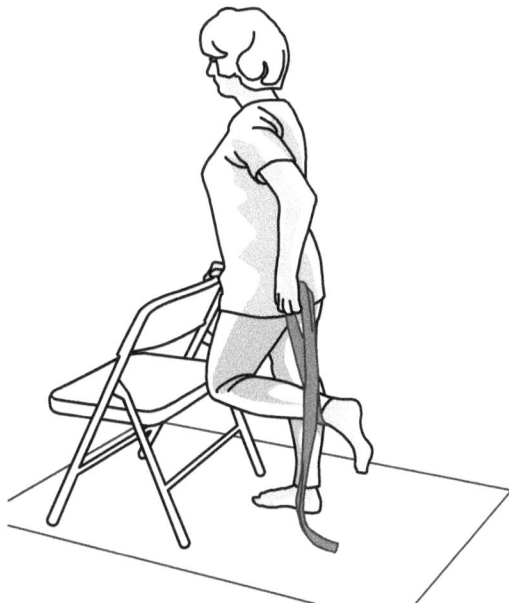

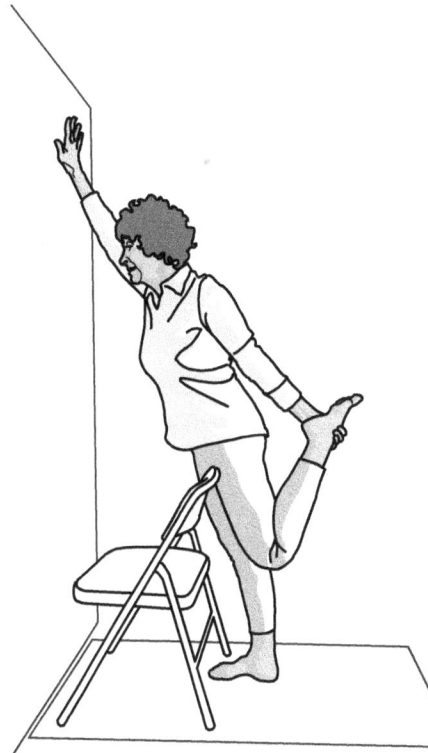

Restorative

Uttanasana (Forward Fold) Bow-to-Grace with Two Chairs (p. 69)

Hold for five to ten minutes.

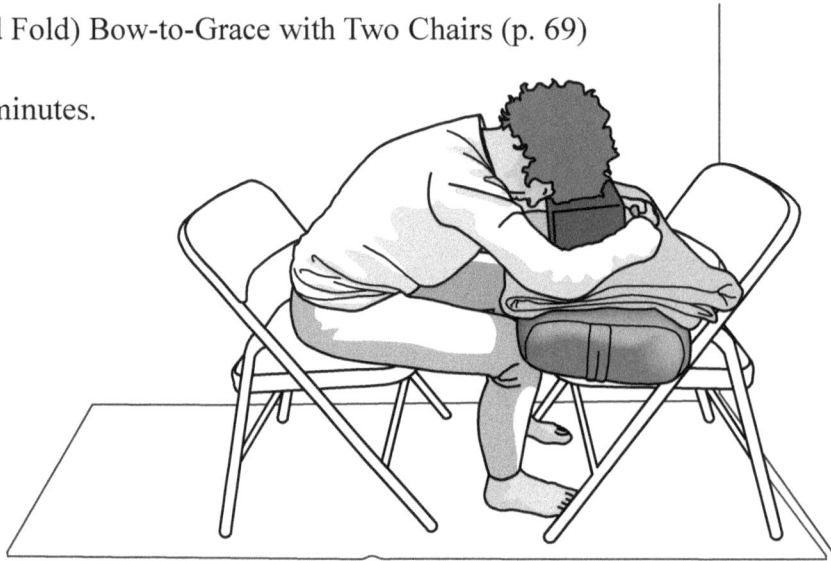

Savasana

Cozy Lying-Down Savasana with Props (p. 76)

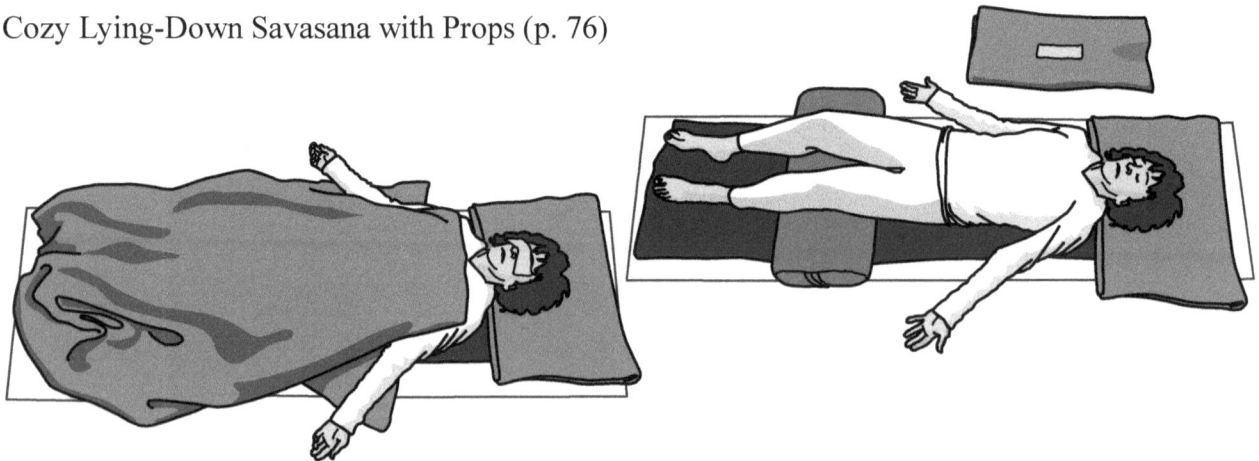

Closing Your Practice (p. 79)

Design-Your-Own Sequence: Total Body (60-min & 30-min)

Listening to the body means to respect its limitations, to let go of the ego when deciding how deep or long to hold any pose, or how long or often to practice, or which poses to practice. Listen to your body as you experiment below with the myriad asanas you can sequence for a complete sixty-minute or thirty-minute practice.

Gather all the props needed for the asanas you select and have them close by for easy access.

For a one-hour practice:
1. Observe the breath and set an intention (p. 7).
2. Optional: Choose one mudra from Chapter II (pp. 11–12).
3. Optional: Choose one mantra from Chapter II (pp. 12–13).
4. Choose one pranayama from Chapter II (pp. 6–11).
5. Choose two asanas from each of the seven sections in Chapter III (pp. 21–63).
6. Choose one asana from Chapter IV (pp. 65–73).
7. Choose one asana from Chapter V (pp. 75–79).
8. Close your practice (p. 79).

For a thirty-minute practice:
1. Observe the breath and set an intention (p. 7).
2. Optional: Choose one mudra from Chapter II (pp. 11–12).
3. Optional: Choose one mantra from Chapter II (pp. 12–13).
4. Choose one pranayama from Chapter II (pp. 6–11).
5. Choose one asana from Chapter III (pp. 21–63).
6. Choose one asana from Chapter IV (pp. 65–73).
7. Choose one asana from Chapter V (pp. 75–79).
8. Close your practice (p. 79).

If your body needs localized stretching or relaxation, select asanas (or additional asanas) for the targeted area; if your body needs rest or recovery, select more restorative asanas or fewer asanas total, and avoid asanas that may aggravate an existing injury. Trust yourself to know what will heal and refresh your body, heart, and soul.

Precaution: If you are pregnant or have high blood pressure or glaucoma, consult your doctor before adding inversions to your sequence—poses in which the heart is higher from the ground than the head.

Whether you follow one of the sample Healing Chair Yoga sequences or design your own, be creative and enjoy your practice! Yoga is, ultimately, the cultivation of self-awareness and self-love. If you feel discomfort or pain, physical or emotional, you are not practicing yoga. Yoga is surrender, letting go, melting into the poses. Yoga is truly a journey to your divine self.

I bow to all of you for being courageous as you begin or renew your yoga practice. The light in me sees the light in you. Namaste.

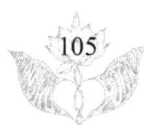

There are only two mistakes one can make along the road to truth:
not going all the way and not starting.
~attributed to the Buddha, Siddhartha Gautama

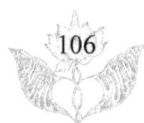

About the Author

Linda Anastasia Ransom, LPC, E-RYT 500, YACEP, C-IAYT, began exploring yoga in 1994, to improve her health and stress management. In 2002, she suffered from a stroke; in 2003, she recovered from it. In 2009, she was diagnosed with breast cancer; in 2010, she was cancer-free and remains so to this day. Linda attributes her swift recovery from both to hard work, her fervent dedication to life, her embracing of disease, her expanding love of her body, and yoga, especially the practices of pranayama (breathing) and dhyana (meditation), which strengthened her presence and mindfulness. Yoga is the life-force energy that has helped her grow mentally, physically, emotionally, and spiritually.

Linda has been teaching yoga since 2005, completing her 200-hour and 500-hour trainings in Iyengar-style Hatha yoga, with Lynne Minton, at Inner Dance Yoga Studio, in Anchorage, Alaska. In 2009, she opened The Anjali Yoga Room to bring the heart of yoga to her home community of Wasilla, Alaska. Through 2021, when it closed mid-pandemic, Linda's studio offered many styles of yoga—Hatha, Vinyasa, hot yoga, pre-natal yoga, core yoga, Yoga for Healing, and Healing Chair Yoga (HCY), including HCY for cancer—with a commitment to honor, in a supportive, loving environment, all individuals with reverence, in their pursuit of health and wellness. The Anjali Yoga Room also hosted yoga-teacher trainings (200-hour with Karen and Bruce Greenwood, 500-hour with Donna and Jeff Martens), and was the first studio in Alaska to certify 500-hour yoga therapists, inviting many outstanding yogis to share their knowledge. Linda maintains a leadership role in the yoga community, providing guidance for others endeavoring to open their own studios.

Because yoga has resonated wholeheartedly in her life, Linda earned, in 2017, her certification as a Yoga Therapist (C-IAYT) through the International Association of Yoga Therapists. She incorporates breathwork, meditation, mindfulness, mantras, mudras, and stress-reduction techniques into her mental health practice as a Licensed Professional Counselor (LPC) at The Wellness Center she founded in 2003. Individuals are empowered to work on self-discovery to release depression, anxiety, stress, and trauma. Linda continues to grow with every student/client she encounters. She reminds us that the real healer is you!

Linda came to Alaska in 1978 to attend the University of Fairbanks. Her devotion to yoga and wholistic health follows a 24-year career in Alaska's public schools as a teacher and a counselor. She has lived in Wasilla since 1989, currently sharing a log home on Wasilla Lake, surrounded by the Chugach Mountains, with her husband of 34 years, Bob; her son, Nico; her future daughter-in-law, Nikki; and her dog, Dave.

To connect with Linda, email her at healingchairyoga@gmail.com.

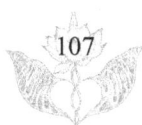

www.ingramcontent.com/pod-product-compliance
Lightning Source LLC
Chambersburg PA
CBHW042339030426
42335CB00030B/3399